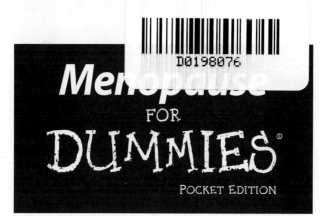

Menopause
FOR
DUMMIES®
POCKET EDITION

by Marcia L. Jones, PhD

Contributing author
Theresa Eichenwald, MD

Look for Pocket Editions on these other topics:

Allergies For Dummies, Pocket Edition
Anxiety & Depression For Dummies, Pocket Edition
Asthma For Dummies, Pocket Edition
Diabetes For Dummies, Pocket Edition
Dieting For Dummies, Pocket Edition
Heart Disease For Dummies, Pocket Edition
High Blood Pressure For Dummies, Pocket Edition
Migraines For Dummies, Pocket Edition

WILEY

Wiley Publishing, Inc.

Menopause For Dummies® Pocket Edition

Published by
Wiley Publishing, Inc.
111 River St.
Hoboken, NJ 07030-5774
www.wiley.com

For general information on our other products and services, please contact our Customer Care Department within the U.S. at 800-762-2974, outside the U.S. at 317-572-3993, or fax 317-572-4002.

For technical support, please visit www.wiley.com/techsupport.

Wiley also publishes its books in a variety of electronic formats. Some content that appears in print may not be available in electronic books.

Library of Congress Control Number: 2005936649

ISBN-13: 978-0-471-79235-2

ISBN-10: 0-471-79235-7

Manufactured in the United States of America

10 9 8 7 6 5 4 3 2 1

1O/RT/QR/QW/IN

Publisher's Acknowledgements

Editor: Elizabeth Kuball
Composition Services: Indianapolis Composition Services Department
Cover Photo: © Stephen Simpson/Getty Images/FPG

Table of Contents

Introduction

• •

*W*e wrote this book to give women of all ages a clear view of the physical, mental, and emotional changes related to menopause. For generations, women of all ages have wandered blindly into menopause without knowing what to expect. Oh, you probably knew that menopause and hot flashes go hand in hand, but even that information isn't always true. The truth is that you may never have a hot flash, and if you do, it will probably be years before you're menopausal. Common knowledge about menopause is sparse and often wrong. (The medical community didn't even officially recognize the link between estrogen and hot flashes until 1974!)

If menopause only concerned a small group of people on a desert island, this lack of information might be understandable. But over half of the world's population will become menopausal one day.

Menopause has been the ugly family member of the research community for years. Even medical textbooks pay scant attention to the topic. Today, one group is paying attention to menopause: The pharmaceutical industry sees great opportunity in the field of menopause, and more research is underway.

If you're looking for books to help reasonably intelligent women navigate the jungle of menopause (menopause is uncharted territory), your options are largely limited to pretty, glossy pamphlets published by drug companies (now that's what we call unbiased information) that you can find at your doctor's office. If you're really persistent, you may find some academic articles in medical journals, but your eyes will glass over as you try to pick out straightforward answers to your practical questions.

We hope this book can fill that void. Our goal is to help you digest the research so you can make better and objective health decisions.

Menopause is not a medical condition — that's true. No one is going to die from menopause or its symptoms, but every day, women die from the medical effects of low estrogen levels. Your risks of certain diseases and cancers rise after menopause. Some folks may respond to that statement with one of their own, "Well, that's because women are older when they go through menopause." True again, but it's also true that estrogen plays a role in an amazing number of functions in your body, some of which protect your organs, increase your immunity, and slow degeneration. This transformation we call menopause impacts our health in very significant ways. This book helps you understand the story behind the symptoms and the diseases.

Some women choose to use hormone therapy to relieve symptoms associated with menopause and protect their body from disease. The choice of whether to take hormones or not is quite controversial because hormone therapy has its own set of risks. The debate goes on in the medical community and media concerning the risks of hormone therapy. If you're like many women, your confusion only grows as you read more on the subject. Each new study seems to contradict the findings of the last one. You're an intelligent person. But how can you know which study you should believe? In this book, we try to provide enough information to enable you to make informed decisions about your health.

About This Book

We have no agenda in writing this book. We're not trying to sell you medications, alternative health strategies, or remedies. This book presents accurate and up-to-date information from the most credible sources. It contains straightforward information based on reliable medical studies without the academic lingo common to medical journals. When no clear-cut answers exist and when quality research shows mixed conclusions, we let you know.

We know your life is busy, so we cut to the chase. We cover the questions that are important to you during this phase of your life. We also try not to stray too far from the topic at hand. For example, during the years leading up to menopause, women may have difficulty getting pregnant. The same hormonal changes that cause those annoying symptoms prior to menopause also stifle fertility. Many women in their late 30s who are trying to get pregnant rely on hormone supplements. Despite the overlap in hormonal terms, fertility is not a concern for many women going through the change, so our discussion is limited.

Whether you're going through the change, have already been there, or are about to start off down that road, you'll find the information you need between these snazzy yellow-and-black covers.

Foolish Assumptions

Every author has to make a few assumptions about her audience, and we've made a few assumptions about you:

✔ **You're a woman.** Sorry, guys, but menopause is a girls-only club.

✔ **You want to understand what's going on with your body.**

✔ **You're looking for straight talk for real people as opposed to scientific jargon and Medicalese.** That said, we have a Medicalese icon to warn you when we stray into this territory (see "Icons Used in This Book," later in this Introduction).

✔ **You want to evaluate your risks of disease as you pass through midlife and move into your menopausal years.**

✔ **You don't want a book that claims to let you diagnose yourself or figure out what medications you need.** You have a medical advisor to discuss these things with.

✔ **You want to be able to ask intelligent questions and discuss treatment alternatives with your healthcare providers.**

✔ **You want to feel more confident about the quality of your healthcare.**

✔ **You buy every book that has a black and yellow cover.**

If any of these statements applies to you, you're in the right place.

Conventions Used in This Book

As you read this book, you'll discover that menopause is a process, with different stages characterized by similar symptoms. These stages are

✔ **Perimenopause,** the three to ten years prior to menopause when you may experience symptoms.

✔ *Menopause* itself, which you know you've reached only after you've reached it because the definition of menopause is the absence of periods for a year.

✔ *Postmenopause,* which is your life after you've stopped having periods. In this book, we use *perimenopause* to describe the premenopause condition, and we use *menopause* to refer to everything after that just because the term *post-menopause* isn't commonly used.

A major part of this book — Chapters 3, 4, 5, and 6 — talks about hormone therapy (HT), which is used to alleviate symptoms and address health concerns prompted by menopause. In literature and on Web sites, you can see hormone therapies referred to and abbreviated any number of ways, including hormone replacement therapy (HRT) and estrogen replacement therapy (ERT). But we stick pretty closely to using HT because we feel that it's the most inclusive and accurate term. Just be aware that *HT* means essentially the same thing as *HRT.*

And, speaking of hormones, a couple of the more important ones for menopausal women have several subcategories:

✔ Types of **estrogen** include estriol, estradiol, and estrone.

✔ **Progesterone** is the class of hormone; the form used in hormone therapy is often referred to as progestin.

We sometimes use these terms interchangeably and only refer to the specific hormone as necessary for clarity.

Icons Used in This Book

In this book, we use icons as a quick way to go directly to the information you need. Look for the icons in the margin that point out specific types of information. Here's what the icons we use in this book mean.

 The Tip icon points out practical, concise information that can help you take better care of yourself.

 This icon points you to medical terms and jargon that can help you understand what you read or hear from professionals and enables you to ask your healthcare provider intelligent questions.

 This fine piece of art flags information that's worth noting.

 When you see this icon, do what it tells you to do. It accompanies info that you should discuss with an expert in the field.

 The Technical Stuff icon points out material that generally can be classified as dry as a bone. Although we think that the information is interesting, it's not vital to your understanding of the issue. Skip it if you so desire.

 This icon cautions you about potential problems or threats to your health.

Where to Go from Here

For Dummies books are designed so that you can dip in anywhere that looks interesting and get the information you need. This is a reference book, so don't feel like you have to read an entire chapter (or even an entire section for that matter). You won't miss anything by skipping around. So, find what interests you and jump on in!

If you want even more information on menopause, from the nitty-gritty of what menopause does to your mind and body, to fitness programs that are great for menopausal women, check out the full-size version of *Menopause For Dummies* — simply head to your local book seller or go to www.dummies.com!

Chapter 1

Reversing Puberty

. . . .

In This Chapter

▶ Getting your feet wet with the basics on menopause

▶ Figuring out where you are on the menopausal roadmap

▶ Understanding the symptoms

▶ Outlining healthcare options

▶ Living a long and healthy life

. . . .

"**Y**ou've come a long way, baby" seems like a recurring slogan for Baby Boomers. The phrase certainly says a lot about the women of this generation as they approach the rite of passage we call menopause. As an individual, you no doubt feel as though you've come a long way in your life by the time you begin to think about menopause. Society, in general, and women, in particular, have also come a long way in opening up the discussion about the mysteries of menopause.

Puberty and menopause bracket the reproductive season of your life, and they share many characteristics. Both puberty and menopause are transitions (meaning that they don't last forever), they're both triggered by hormones, and they both cause physical and emotional changes (that sometimes drive you crazy).

Puberty was the time when your hormones first swung into action. It marked the beginning of your reproductive years. Remember the ride? Your hormone levels shifted wildly and caused your first menstrual period. And don't forget the erratic emotions — what we like to call the teenage crazies. Over the course of a few years, your hormones found a comfortable level. Your unpredictable periods finally settled into a predictable pattern, and your emotional balance was more or less restored.

At the end of your reproductive years, your hormone levels go through a similar dance (this time causing the midlife crazies), but your hormones eventually find a new, lower level of production. Your periods are erratic for a while, but they eventually wind down and stop. Just in case you're wondering, those midlife emotional crazies eventually pass, too.

Keep in mind that the phrase "you've come a long way, baby" closes with "but you've got such a long way to go." Women today often live 40 or 50 years after menopause. We all want to enjoy these years by visiting friends, taking care of our loved ones and ourselves, and continuing to participate in activities that give us pleasure.

In this chapter, we introduce you to menopause so you know what to expect when the time comes or what has been happening to you if you're already in transition.

Defining Menopause

Have you ever noticed how you don't really pay close attention to directions or where you're going when you're the passenger in a car? You only start to worry about every exit number and stoplight when you're the one behind the wheel. Well, menopause is like that. We all hear about menopause and menopausal symptoms, but we rarely pay much attention to the particulars until it's our turn.

When you do slide into the driver's seat and start paying attention, you may become frustrated by the confusing terminology associated with the whole menopause thing. Aside from the pamphlets you get from the doctor's office, most books, magazines, and articles treat menopause like a stage that starts with hot flashes and goes on for the rest of your life. But, *menopause* actually means the end of menstruation. During the years leading up to menopause (called *perimenopause*), your periods may be so erratic that you're never sure which period will be the last one, but you aren't officially menopausal until you haven't had a period for a year.

A lot happens *before* you have your last period, and all this physical and mental commotion is associated with menopause. You may experience hot flashes, mental lapses, mood swings, and heart palpitations while you're still having periods. But, when you ask your doctor if you're menopausal, he or she may check you over and say "no." Relax: Your doctor isn't wrong, and you aren't crazy. You're not menopausal. You're *peri*menopausal.

 Medical folks divide menopause into phases that coincide with physiological changes. We describe these phases in just a second, but you need to know something about the terminology that surrounds menopause. On one hand, you have the medical terms associated with menopause, and on the other, you have the terms that you hear when you're chatting with the girls over coffee or tennis.

The term *perimenopause* refers to the time leading up to the cessation of menstruation, when estrogen production is slowing down. A lot of the symptoms that folks usually label as *menopausal* (hot flashes, mood swings, sleeplessness, and so on) actually take place during the perimenopausal years. We're sticklers in this book about using the term *perimenopause* rather than *menopause* to describe this early phase because you're still having periods. We also use *perimenopause* because we want to note the physiological and emotional changes you experience prior to the end of your periods and distinguish them from the changes that happen after your body has adjusted to lower levels of estrogen.

Technically, the time after your last period is called *postmenopause,* but this word has never really caught on. So, in keeping with common usage, we most often use the term *menopause* to refer to the actual event and the years after menopause and use *postmenopause* only when it helps clarify things. When we talk about *menopausal* women in this book, we're talking about women who have stopped having periods — whether they're 55 or 75.

The years leading up to and following menopause mark a pretty major transformation in a woman's life. As you make your way through this period of your life, you'll want to know where you are within the whole grand scope of the change and what's going on inside you. Here's a brief description of the phases associated with menopause.

Making changes while approaching the change: Perimenopause

Perimenopause is the stage during which your hormones start to change gears. Some months, your hormones operate at the levels they've worked at for the past 30 years or so; other months, your ovaries are tired and don't produce estrogen when they should. Your brain responds to this lack of estrogen production by sending a signal to try to get those ovaries jumpstarted. When they receive the signal, your ovaries leap out of bed and overcompensate for their laziness by producing double or triple the normal amount of estrogen.

Your period is late because your ovaries were dozing during the first part of your normal cycle. Your period is super-heavy because, when your ovaries wake up, they overcompensate by producing way too much estrogen (just as, after you wake up having slept through your alarm, you may run around like a chicken with its head cut off).

So, during perimenopause, you still have your period, but you experience symptoms that folks associate with menopause. If you go to the doctor at this stage and ask, "What's happening to me? Could this be menopause?" the doctor will often go straight to the "Could this be menopause?" part of your question. Of course, you're not menopausal if you're still having periods. But the problem is that many doctors miss the first part of the question — the "What's happening to me?" part. This is the real issue you want to get to the bottom of — the cause of your weird physical and emotional conditions.

Menstruating no more: To menopause and beyond

Menopause means never having to say, "Can I borrow a tampon?" again.

If you haven't had a period for a year, you've reached *menopause*. Women can become menopausal approximately any time between the ages of 45 and 55, with the average age being 51. The definition may seem cut and dried at first glance, but here are a few situations that may leave you scratching your head.

What if you use a cyclical type of hormone therapy in which you take estrogen for several days and progestin during the last few days of your cycle? You still have a period (the progestin causes you to slough the lining of the uterus), but you don't ovulate. Are you menopausal or not? Technically, you're delaying your last period. You're taking a sufficient dosage of estrogen to rid yourself of perimenopausal symptoms, but you're no longer fertile.

Here's another tricky one: If you've had a *hysterectomy* (surgical removal of the uterus), you're menopausal according to the basic definition. But, if you had your uterus removed but kept your ovaries, you're not "hormonally" menopausal because your ovaries still produce estrogen. By taking your blood and analyzing your hormone levels, your physician can tell you whether your hormones are officially at menopausal levels.

These tricky situations cause us to ask, "Who cares about the definition?" You know a rose is a rose. The main concern here is *what's happening with your hormones,* especially estrogen. Hormonal changes can trigger many physical and emotional health issues.

When you reach menopause, your hormone production is so low that your periods stop. Your ovaries still produce some estrogen and testosterone, but instead of producing hormones in cycles (which is why you have periods and why you're only fertile for about four or five days each month), your body now produces constant, low levels of hormones. The type of estrogen your ovaries churn out also switches from an active type to a rather inactive form.

Postmenopause is the period of your life that starts after menopause (a year after your last period) and ends when you do. This is a time when your body is living on greatly reduced levels of estrogen, testosterone, and progesterone. In this book, we simply refer to both the cessation of your period and your life afterwards as menopause.

Anticipating Menopause

When will you become menopausal? The timing varies from woman to woman. Predicting this stuff is nowhere near an exact science. Heck, you can't even use the fact that you started your period earlier than most women as a predictor that you'll stop menstruating earlier. (The same goes for starting your period later in life and ending it later in life.) Genetics and lifestyle may have some impact on the schedule, but basically, it happens when it happens. However, we can give you some ballpark age ranges for these phases.

Most women become perimenopausal sometime between the ages of 35 and 50. You'll probably know it when you get there because you'll probably have some of the symptoms (check out Chapter 2) and/or some irregular periods. Women usually become menopausal sometime in their 50s.

Men-o-pause

When men experience mood swings and mental lapses during their 50s, they (or you) may think that they're going through the change, too. But the change men go through is quite different from the one women experience.

The rise and fall of hormones in a woman's body follows a cyclical pattern. Hormone levels shift throughout the month on a regular basis. So, every 28 to 35 days, a woman has the chance to become pregnant. The hormonal changes prepare her body for conception and pregnancy.

Men have no cycle (besides, perhaps, the yearly cycle based on the presence or absence of football in their systems). Their primary sex hormone, testosterone, stays at a fairly constant level from day to day, so men don't experience cyclical fluctuations. But men's testosterone levels do decline with age. Lower testosterone levels generally result in lower libido (sex drive) in males and generally occur when men are in their late 50s or 60s.

Do men go through menopause? There's no question that the decline of sex hormones in men results in lower libido, weaker bones, and an increased risk of prostate cancer. But the changes are simply a result of the natural aging process and are not triggered by a change in hormonal patterns.

Some events can alter these "normal" age patterns, including lifestyle habits and medical interventions. Here are a few exceptional types of menopause:

✔ **Premature menopause:** A term used when women go through menopause in their thirties. This timing is considered unusually early, but it may be normal for you.

- ✔ **Medical menopause:** Refers to menopause induced by chemotherapy or radiation therapy. Sometimes these treatments can cause a pause in your body's normal cycle. However, this type of menopause is often reversed after treatments are finished, though your periods may take a month, several months, or even years to return.

- ✔ **Surgical menopause:** Refers to menopause induced by surgery. Removal of both ovaries results in immediate, nonreversible menopause. Because your ovaries produce all types of sex hormones (estrogen, progesterone, and testos-terone), surgical removal of your ovaries is fairly traumatic for your system, and you typi-cally experience intense perimenopausal symp-toms (hot flashes and the like).

 Excessive exercising or an eating disorder can cause a temporary halt in your periods (a condi-tion called *amenorrhea*), but your periods will return to normal when your lifestyle returns to normal. This is not menopause but rather a medical condition that needs to be treated.

Experiencing Menopause

When women talk about their personal experiences of puberty, menstrual cycles, and pregnancy, the stories are all over the board. Some women don't notice changes in their bodies; others recognize the moment ovulation or conception occurs. Some women have terrible problems with premenstrual syndrome (PMS); others have trouble-free cycles throughout their entire lives. Women's experiences vary with perimenopause and menopause just as much as they vary with these other changes.

Identifying symptoms

Less than half of all women experience annoying symptoms such as hot flashes, heart palpitations, interrupted sleep, and mood swings during the transition period prior to menopause. Most women who do experience these symptoms experience the symptoms while they're still menstruating on a regular schedule.

Other women recognize that they're perimenopausal because their periods, which used to be as regular as clockwork, are now irregular. Their periods may be late, they may skip a period, or their flow may be light one month and resemble a flood the next month.

Unfortunately, no objective medical test exists to determine whether you're officially perimenopausal.

We devote Chapter 2 almost exclusively to the symptoms women may experience during perimenopause.

Calling in the professionals

If you're in your late 40s or 50s and you're experiencing the symptoms listed in Chapter 2, you can probably assume that you're peri-menopausal. But don't cancel that appointment with your medical advisor to get the symptoms checked out. (If you don't have an appointment to cancel, make one and keep it.) Many symptoms of perimenopause are the same as some of the symptoms of thyroid problems, cardiovascular disease, depression, and other serious health issues.

Your medical practitioner can help you deal with the undesirable symptoms of perimenopause and prevent serious health conditions that are more prevalent after menopause.

Making Time for Menopause

You may be wondering when the perimenopause and menopause phase of your life will hit and how long the symptoms will last.

Starting out

Most women's ovaries begin a transformation some-time between the ages of 35 and 50. If you start the change before you reach 40, you experience what's known as *premature menopause.*

Perimenopause is sometimes called a *climacteric period,* which simply means that it's a crucial period. Remember that your ovaries don't just shut down one day; the transition is punctuated with production peaks and valleys that cause many annoying physical and mental symptoms. Perimenopause is a time of important physiological change — when egg production slows along with the production of estrogen and progesterone begins slowing down.

Seeing it through to the end

Because you never really know when perimenopause starts, accurately defining a timeframe is difficult. Some women experience symptoms for ten years before their periods stop. The fact is that most of the symptoms you hear about are caused by the fluctuating hormone levels of perimenopause as opposed to the sustained, low levels of hormones you experience during menopause.

You're officially menopausal one year after your last period. After that, many people use the term *post-menopause* to mark the rest of your life (though in this book, we just keep using the word *menopause*).

Treating Menopause

At the end of the perimenopause road, your ovaries (and consequently, your hormone production) finally wind down. Your body gradually adjusts to the lower hormone levels typical of life after menopause. Most of the perimenopausal symptoms disappear, but now your concerns shift to health issues associated with prolonged, lowered levels of active estrogen.

Estrogen not only plays a role in reproduction, it also helps regulate a host of other functions throughout your body. Estrogen protects your bones and cardiovascular system, among other responsibilities. Those pesky perimenopausal symptoms may make life miserable, but they aren't dangerous to your health. But the conditions associated with long periods of diminished estrogen levels are very troublesome. They include

- ✔ Cardiovascular disease
- ✔ Heart disease
- ✔ Hypertension (high blood pressure)
- ✔ Osteoporosis
- ✔ Stroke

So you and your doctor need to work on strategies to prevent these conditions.

Some women choose hormone therapy (HT) to help prevent disease; others choose to take medications as individual problems arise. (We cover hormone therapy in Chapters 3 and 4 and non-hormonal ways to deal with certain conditions in Chapters 5 and 6.) Some women try alternatives to traditional medicine such as herbs or acupuncture (check out Chapter 5). Whichever path or paths you choose, each strategy presents benefits and risks. Your choices depend on your medical history, your family history, and your healthcare preferences. And remember that both your experiences and medical technologies change daily, so reevaluate your options from time to time.

Promoting Longevity

Not long ago, 50 was about as old as people could expect to get. Today, many people live well into their 70s, 80s, and 90s. The fact that most women stop being fertile in their 40s doesn't mean that women are no longer productive after 40. In fact, with the whole reproduction thing out of the way, women have more time and opportunities to make new contributions to life on Earth (or in space).

One of the keys to a long and happy life is good genes. Another key is taking good care of yourself and the genes you're dealt. Regular checkups can address medical issues as they arise and help prevent others. Eat healthy foods (and portions), get some exercise, and live life to its fullest.

Everyone agrees that a healthy lifestyle is the best way to reduce troublesome perimenopausal symptoms, prevent disease, and promote a long and healthy life. It's also the least risky strategy for dealing with perimenopause and menopause. Taking up this challenge requires self-assessment and a bit of determination. Shifting to a healthy lifestyle involves eliminating unhealthy habits, getting at least a half-hour of aerobic exercise five times a week, and maintaining a healthy, balanced diet that includes at least five servings of fruit and vegetables each week.

Chapter 2

Getting in Sync with the Symptoms

• •

In This Chapter

▶ Getting in touch with the changes before the change

▶ Discovering the physical and emotional effects of menopause

▶ Talking to your doctor

• •

*Y*ou're irritable for no reason, you have trouble sleeping, you experience heart palpitations, and your sex drive is getting a little crazy. Sound familiar? If so, you're almost certainly starting down the road to menopause.

Every human body is unique — that's no surprise. But the path to menopause reveals just how different we really are. Some women breeze through the change, experiencing very few physical or emotional indications that anything is happening. Other women experience disturbing symptoms for an extended period of time. Fortunately, the symptoms often pass as you move into menopause and beyond.

In this chapter, we provide an introduction to the perimenopausal and menopausal symptoms you may experience.

The symptoms we discuss in this chapter are all symptoms of perimenopause or menopause, but they're not unique to perimenopause and menopause. Other medical conditions cause these symptoms as well. If you experience any of these symptoms, don't just assume that they're a result of perimenopause or menopause. Your doctor will want to check out other possible causes.

Kicking Things Off with Perimenopausal Symptoms

In this section, we give you the laundry list of symptoms that have been attributed to the sudden drops of estrogen during perimenopause. Women experience none, a few, or quite a few of these symptoms to greater or lesser degrees. If you think we sound wishy-washy, we're guilty as charged, but we have to hedge our bets because each person is unique.

If you have yet to experience perimenopause or menopause, you can take heart in the following statistic, but if you're currently experiencing symptoms you may want to hide this statistic from the folks you live with: Only 40 to 60 percent of women in the United States report experiencing any perimenopausal symptoms. For women who do experience symptoms, the symptoms can range in severity from being somewhat annoying to interfering with their ability to enjoy life.

Getting physical

When you heard Olivia Newton-John belt out "Let's get physical" a million years ago, did you ever think that it would come down to this? We surely didn't, but it has, so we need to outline the physical side of perimenopause — as in the outward, physical signs that your body's hormones are a-changing.

Many of the physical symptoms are the result of a string of events that happens when *estradiol* (the active form of estrogen) levels suddenly drop — a typical occurrence during perimenopause. The drop causes a chain reaction in your body, which we describe in the "Revealing the biology behind the symptoms" sidebar, later in this chapter.

The relationship between estrogen and serotonin plays a role in many of the mental symptoms, but it also has a hand in some of the physical symptoms — like interrupted sleep. *Serotonin* is a compound that helps the body regulate sleep and moods. Though all the details aren't in, estrogen plays some kind of role in the production and maintenance of serotonin. It's amazing how all this stuff gets connected, huh?

Here are some of the physical symptoms of perimenopause that you may experience:

✔ **Hot flashes:** *Hot flashes* (also called hot flushes) are the traditional, highly recognized symptom of menopause. When you have a hot flash, you suddenly feel very flushed — especially in your face and upper body. Increased perspiration usually accompanies this feeling of warmth. And, sometimes, dizziness, heart palpitations, and a suffocating feeling can precede or accompany hot flashes.

A sudden drop in estrogen levels triggers a hot flash. This drop in estrogen sends a message to your brain that something is terribly wrong, so your brain sends out a power burst of adrenaline (norepinephrine). *Norepinephrine* is the hormone that triggers the fight-or-flight response in humans, so your body moves into ready mode, which gets your blood pressure up, your heart pounding, and also causes the blood vessels in your head, neck, and chest to dilate. All this commotion makes you feel like you're sweltering.

✔ **Night sweats:** *Night sweats* are essentially hot flashes that occur at night. The same estrogen drop that triggers hot flashes during the day triggers night sweats.

Night sweats can also be caused by infection, thyroid problems, or other types of illness, so if this is the only seemingly perimenopausal symptom you experience, check with your doctor.

✔ **Interrupted sleep:** With all the weird symptoms going on during the day, getting a good night's sleep so you can wake up feeling rested doesn't seem like a lot to ask for, but sometimes sleep can be a problem. Hot flashes in the middle of the night often result in interrupted sleep. You wake up, often perspiring (and sometimes cursing), and have a hard time going back to sleep. Interrupted sleep can cause sleep deprivation, which in turn leads to irritability, anxiety, and mood swings.

A rapid drop in estrogen also affects your serotonin levels. Serotonin helps regulate mood and sleep patterns. (Drugs such as Prozac and Zoloft work on the principle that serotonin regulation is key to relieving mood swings, irritability, and so on.) Estrogen makes serotonin more available by prolonging its action. When estrogen drops, it affects your serotonin levels, which contributes to interrupted sleep.

✔ **Heart palpitations:** Butterflies in your stomach often accompany heart flutters, or *palpitations*. The sudden drops in estrogen that are so common during perimenopause cause reactions all over your body (see the "Revealing the biology behind the symptoms" sidebar, later in this chapter), including heart flutters. The drop in estrogen causes your body's natural pain-killers and mood regulators *(endorphins)* to drop. Your body interprets this state of affairs as trouble, so a command is issued to send out a burst of adrenaline (norepinephrine, the fight-or-flight hormone). Your body is responding as though you had just encountered a big grizzly bear. The only trouble is you don't see the grizzly bear, and you're left wondering why your body suddenly decided to get ready to flee from it just when you sat down to a nice candlelit dinner.

✔ **Irregular periods:** Irregular periods are quite common in perimenopausal women because fluctuating hormone levels can interrupt the ovulation cycle. Some months you ovulate; some months you don't. If you don't ovulate, you don't produce enough progesterone to have a period, so the lining of your uterus builds up.

✔ **Heavy bleeding:** Heavy bleeding during perimenopause is usually caused by an "eggless" cycle. You make estrogen during the first part of your cycle, but for some reason (often unknown), you just don't ovulate. Therefore, you don't produce progesterone, and you develop an unusually thick uterine lining, which you shed during your period. This process translates into abnormally heavy bleeding.

✔ **Headaches:** For women who experience intense headaches during the first few days of their periods, we have some bad news — you may have more headaches during perimenopause. Headaches during the first few days of your period mean that you're sensitive to low estrogen levels, which are typical at that time. When estrogen levels drop quickly, which happens during perimenopause, the drop may trigger another one of those headaches.

✔ **Fibroids:** *Fibroids* are simply balls of uterine muscle tissue. Nearly one-third of women have fibroids by the time they're 50. Fibroids tend to get bigger as you approach menopause, but they usually don't grow in size after menopause. You really don't need to do anything about fibroids unless they cause symptoms such as pain, pressure, or increased bleeding.

The approach to menopause can be blamed for a number of menstrual irregularities. But remember that you can't blame all irregularities on perimenopause. Although the menstrual symptoms we list above (irregular periods and heavy bleeding) often wait for women on the road to the change, consult your healthcare provider about these and all other symptoms before simply writing them off to peri-menopause.

Playing head games

The mental/emotional symptoms associated with per-imenopause can be very frustrating given that many women don't associate their recent irritability or depression with perimenopause.

The symptoms we list generally pass after your hormones settle into their new, lower levels after menopause. However, these symptoms severely inconvenience or otherwise bother many women during perimenopause. If this description mirrors your situation, there's no need sit there suffering in silence.

✔ **Mood swings:** Mood swings are common among perimenopausal women. But remember that mood swings are also common before your period (part of premenstrual syndrome) and after pregnancy. Although medical researchers

Revealing the biology behind the symptoms

As you may have suspected, the symptoms of menopause are all tied to plunging hormone levels. You may feel these symptoms more frequently during perimenopause than menopause because your hormone levels fluctuate more during perimenopause. Sometimes they rise to fairly normal levels, and then they come crashing down. The *fluctuation* is the trigger for a lot of the symptoms. In menopause, hormone levels are consistently lower than they are during your reproductive years, so they don't pop up and drop down so frequently, though symptoms can still occur.

Here's a step-by-step guide of what happens to your body when your estradiol (the active form of estrogen) levels drop:

1. Your ovaries produce lower levels of estradiol, which causes a drop in the amount of estradiol reaching the brain.

2. Less estradiol in the brain causes a decrease in your endorphin levels. *Endorphins* are your body's natural painkillers and mood regulators. (If you're a runner, you're probably familiar with the effects of endorphins — they cause the "runner's high.")

3. Lower levels of endorphins in your brain cause it to think that something is terribly wrong, so it sends out a burst of adrenaline, namely *norepinephrine* (the hormone that triggers the fight-or-flight response).

4. The burst of norepinephrine causes your body to kick into ready-for-anything mode by increasing your heart rate (which causes those palpitations and flutters), raising your blood pressure, and dilating your blood vessels. Dilating blood vessels cause the hot flashes and sweating. If you're asleep, you may wake up suddenly. You may also experience diarrhea or get a feeling of anxiety and butterflies in your stomach.

don't know all the details, low levels of estrogen are associated with lower levels of serotonin, which can lead to mood swings, in addition to irritability, anxiety, pain sensitivity, eating disorders, and insomnia.

✓ **Anxiety:** Anxiety is another common symptom perimenopausal women face. Like mood swings, anxiety seems to be tied to low levels of estrogen. The lower levels of endorphins and serotonin associated with low estrogen levels may trigger anxiety. Another theory is that low levels of estrogen, serotonin, and endorphins leave you more susceptible to the emotional stressors in your world. With this theory, lower estrogen, serotonin, and endorphin levels don't trigger anxiety; they simply inhibit your ability to easily deal with stressful situations.

✓ **Irritability:** The same hormonal shifts that cause mood swings and anxiety cause irritability. Like these other symptoms, irritability is a temporary condition that seems to blow over after you're menopausal (if you can put up with yourself for that long).

✓ **Memory problems:** Memory problems during perimenopause sneak up on you. You forget your friend's name one day; you leave your keys somewhere in the grocery store another day. Pretty soon you start remembering how many times you couldn't remember something. We're not talking about dementia or Alzheimer's disease here; we're talking about forgetfulness and a lack of focus. This category covers relatively minor memory glitches: You forget where you're going with a thought in mid-sentence, or you get to the store and forget what you need to buy Thank goodness for sticky notes and grocery lists.

Estrogen seems to facilitate communication among *neurons* (nerve cells) in the brain. Much of memory is a matter of the brain sending information from one memory storage center to another. Because estrogen helps maintain connections and grow new ones, shifting estrogen levels can stymie communication between memory storage areas. Memory problems seem to be a short-term issue; some women seem to lose the memory lapses after menopause.

We still don't know if hormones have anything to do with more permanent types of dementia or Alzheimer's disease. But the research is pointing in the direction that says estrogen could reduce the risk (or at least slow down the progression) of the Alzheimer's disease later in life.

✔ **Fuzzy thinking:** Fuzzy thinking is common when you're deprived of sleep or your hormones are in flux. When we say *fuzzy thinking*, we mean the feeling that you're just not with it today — like you're walking through a fog or you just can't concentrate on what you're doing. Fuzzy thinking can be the result of interrupted sleep (which isn't uncommon during perimenopause).

Fluctuating hormone levels also cause fuzzy thinking (as you may have experienced during pregnancy or at certain points in your menstrual cycle). Like many of the symptoms that accompany perimenopause, this too shall pass. Fuzzy thinking is a temporary thing. It generally clears up when your hormones settle down and your sleep patterns chill out during menopause.

Be sure to inform your medical professional about these mental and emotional symptoms. They may be more closely related to hormonal imbalances than to psychological issues. But, either way, your healthcare professional can ensure that you get the proper treatment to alleviate your symptoms.

Visiting the Menopausal Symptoms

All the symptoms we describe as *perimenopausal* have long been attributed to menopause. But after you're menopausal (without a menstrual period for a year), things begin to settle down a bit. Hot flashes subside and your moods stabilize. Your body and psyche seem to get used to some aspects of lower estrogen production.

The symptoms experienced after menopause are sometimes a bit more uncomfortable physically.

 Long periods of low levels of estrogen encourage conditions such as osteoporosis, cardiovascular disease, heart attack, stroke, colon cancer, and other diseases.

 To avoid wordiness, we use the term *menopause* in this chapter (and most others) to refer to the time period that incorporates both menopause and postmenopause.

Figuring out the physical facts

After your ovaries retire (well, they never really retire — they just greatly reduce their workload), you produce lower levels of estrogen without the sudden spikes and drops typical of perimenopause. Your hormones calm down — way down. As time goes by, these long periods of low estrogen levels result in some physical changes. In this section, we discuss what these conditions feel like.

Some of the symptoms are the result of lower levels of estrogen, pure and simple. We call these *primary symptoms*. Some of these primary symptoms can actually cause further unpleasantness, which we call *secondary symptoms*.

The primary symptoms include

- ✔ **Vaginal dryness:** The medical establishment refers to this condition as *vaginal atrophy*. Because estrogen keeps vaginal tissues moisturized and pliant, continuous periods of low estrogen can result in the drying out and shrinking of vaginal tissue. Between 20 and 45 percent of women in the United States experience vaginal dryness. They often notice it when intercourse becomes painful due to a lack of lubrication.

- ✔ **Vulvar discomfort:** Itching, burning, and dryness of the vulva isn't uncommon among menopausal women. But remember that many conditions and diseases that affect the vulva have nothing to do with estrogen, so have your doctor check out any vulvar changes.

- ✔ **Urinary incontinence:** This condition is much more prevalent in women after menopause than it is during the reproductive years. The tissues of your urinary tract become drier and thinner, and the muscles lose their tone as estrogen levels diminish. You know you're experiencing urinary incontinence if you have a hard time holding it when you laugh, exercise, or sneeze. Your urinary tract, especially your urethra, depends on estrogen to maintain its form and muscle tone. The urethra has a hard time sealing off the flow of urine after years of diminished estrogen levels.

- ✔ **Urinary frequency:** Like incontinence, urinary frequency results from sustained, low levels of estrogen that define menopause. Urinary frequency simply means that you have to urinate frequently. You may leave the bathroom and quickly feel like you have to go again. This condition can be very frustrating during the day — and even more frustrating at night. Urinary frequency can also cause interrupted sleep, which understandably, turns into irritability.

✔ **Skin changes:** Lower estrogen levels cause your skin to sag and wrinkle. Estrogen doesn't literally prevent sagging. But estrogen does keep your skin elastic and help your skin retain fluid, so it remains "filled out" rather than becoming loose and droopy.

✔ **Hair changes:** Your hair becomes thinner and more brittle with menopause, though some women report that their hair feels as soft and fluffy as cotton several years into menopause. Estrogen seems to be a natural moisturizer, so with lower levels of the stuff flowing through your body, your hair takes a hit and becomes more brittle. You also have a tougher time keeping a perm permanent.

✔ **Weight changes:** Your weight shifts to the center of your body — around your waist. Instead of the lovely pear-shaped body you once had, you take on more of an apple-shaped appearance due to shifting hormone levels. Although you may gain a bit of weight, you probably can't directly blame that on hormonal changes. Your body simply becomes less forgiving about nutritional imbalances and poor eating, drinking, and exercise habits.

It's not over yet. One or more of the primary symptoms can trigger even more unpleasantness. Here you go:

✔ **Painful intercourse:** Experiencing pain during intercourse is generally the result of vaginal dryness or physical changes in the position of the urethra due to changes in the shape of the vagina that happen over time when estrogen levels are continuously low. As low levels of estrogen cause your *urovaginal tissues* (tissues of the vagina and urinary tract) to become thinner and the supporting muscle to lose its tone, your organs naturally shift position a bit.

✔ **Interrupted sleep:** Hot flashes, urinary frequency, anxiety, and a variety of other menopausal symptoms can cause interrupted sleep during the night. You wake up feeling tired and experience fatigue throughout the day because your body isn't able to enter the deep stages of sleep at night.

✔ **Fatigue:** If you consistently don't get a good restful night's sleep or you experience insomnia, you may become fatigued. But fatigue can also be the result of low testosterone levels.

Discovering that it's more than skin deep

The mental/emotional aspects of menopause are more of a mixed bag. Some symptoms experienced during menopause usually decrease or go away completely; others are a bit more difficult to deal with.

✔ **Anxiety:** Often, the anxiety common during perimenopause is caused by the rapid drop in estrogen, which initiates a chain reaction (see the "Revealing the biology behind the symptoms" sidebar in this chapter). After menopause, unexplained anxiety often dies down, and you return to your normal self.

✔ **Depression:** Women who have had hysterectomies are more likely to experience menopause-related depression than women who go through a natural menopause. Researchers don't yet understand why this is the case.

Also, women who have been on estrogen and suddenly quit taking it, rather than going through a weaning process, also have more problems with depression. Estrogen assists in the production of serotonin (a substance that helps regulate moods), so lower levels of estrogen can mean lower levels of serotonin.

✔ **Headaches:** Women who experience their first migraine during perimenopause often find that the migraines go away after menopause.

✔ **Lower libido:** Decreased sex drive is a problem for many menopausal women, but the good news is that 70 percent of women remain sexually active during their perimenopausal and menopausal years. Lower libido can be traced to hormonal imbalances and may be the result of testosterone levels being too low.

✔ **Memory lapses and fuzzy thinking:** Though memory lapses and fuzzy thinking are common during perimenopause, most women notice their concentration and memory return to normal after menopause. Aging can cause mental impairment later in life, but you can't blame everything on menopause!

Unraveling the Mystery

Many people associate the word *symptom* with disease, but the definition we use throughout this book is much closer to the dictionary definition — a condition or event that accompanies something. Sometimes you only see perimenopause in your rearview mirror. You may not know that you experienced perimenopause until years later.

But for many women, perimenopausal symptoms surface at one time or another. If you're like many women, you may feel that weird things keep happening to your body or your emotions. But it may take a little investigation on your part to bring the whole perimenopausal picture into focus.

Maybe you feel a flutter in your chest, and you become convinced that you're on the verge of a heart attack. If you go to a cardiologist to check out heart palpitations, she probably won't even think to check your hormones because she's looking for something in your heart to answer the riddle.

Or maybe the "weird things" going on with you aren't physical at all. Maybe they're emotional — like becoming easily frustrated at work or chewing your kids out 50 times a day for the last two weeks. Many women may think twice about these symptoms, but they don't bring them up with their doctors. If you do mention them to your doctor, she may say something like, "It's nothing." Nothing? We know what you're thinking, "Try telling that to my coworkers and my kids."

After you get a hot flash or two, you may figure out that these "weird things" aren't part of your imagination and that you're getting close to menopause. If you figure out the connection, consider yourself lucky. Few women realize that the heart palpitations and the irritability can be part of the same condition — perimenopause. Having read this book, you can be the local expert — it's up to you to coach other women through this!

Even gynecologists sometimes overlook a hormonal imbalance as the source of symptoms. Women may suspect that their problem is "chemical" or hormonal only to have doctors say that they're too young for menopause or that they're still having periods, so they aren't menopausal.

Some gynecologists go so far as to take a blood test to check your follicle stimulating hormone (FSH) level to rule out menopause. High levels of FSH are indicative of *menopause*. But during perimenopause, your hormone levels go up and down. One month your FSH may be perfectly normal; another month it may be high. Without getting tested month after month, determining whether you're *perimenopausal* is difficult.

But women's estrogen and testosterone levels can (and usually do) get out of whack even before they officially become menopausal, and the imbalance triggers the annoying symptoms often associated with menopause. Sometimes you can become even more frustrated after seeking medical advice because the experts tell you, "It's nothing," or they alarm you with the number and types of tests they want you to take.

The reality is that the symptoms you experience are often more intense before menopause — during perimenopause — than they are after you make the change.

Chapter 3

The Basics
of Hormone Therapy

● ●

In This Chapter

▶ Reviewing the options

▶ Understanding the differences in hormone therapy
regimens

▶ Figuring out the best options for you

● ●

*H*ormone therapy (HT) may not be right for
everyone, but it definitely can relieve many
menopausal symptoms and prevent or postpone diseases that afflict women later in life.

Some women swear by HT, some women fear it, and
some women are currently experimenting with hormone therapy to figure out the types, combinations,
and dosages that are right for them to maximize the
protective effects of HT and minimize the risks.
(Arguments about the potential risks of HT abound,
and we discuss them thoroughly in Chapter 4.)

But many women aren't comfortable enough with
their level of knowledge about HT to make up their
minds about where they stand on the subject. If you're
a member of this group, that's okay. Trying to understand the full significance of the choices presented by

your medical advisors can be frustrating and confusing. In this chapter, we explain the various hormones
and hormone therapy regimens and how they work.

Defining Hormone Therapy

Some experts don't like to include the term *replacement* when referring to hormone therapy because
replacement implies that a *deficiency* exists. Producing
lower levels of hormones isn't a disease; it's one of
many natural, normal transitions a woman's body
makes throughout her lifetime. The simpler and more
accurate term for the hormones prescribed during
perimenopause and menopause is *hormone therapy*.
This term reflects a more progressive attitude about
menopause.

Hormone therapy is a program of estrogen and progestin (both of which are classifications of hormones
that support reproductive functions and other inter-
nal systems), which are administered to relieve perimenopausal and menopausal symptoms and lower
the risk of osteoporosis, colorectal cancer, and perhaps Alzheimer's disease. Doctors often prescribe
hormones during *perimenopause* (the years before
menopause when women experience many of the
symptoms — hot flashes, sleeplessness, and so on —
associated with menopause). After menopause, you
can gradually discontinue use of hormone therapy.

Physicians who recommend hormone therapy after
menopause do so because it protects against osteoporosis and relieves *urogenital atrophy* (thinning and
drying of your vagina or ureter) exacerbated by low
levels of estrogen. In many women, the hormone
boost also improves mood and the sense of well-
being. Some women remain on hormone therapy for
upwards of 20 years; others discontinue use after only

a few years. You and your doctor can work together to determine whether hormone therapy is right for you and how long you should remain on it.

Women without a uterus (women who have had a hysterectomy) may take estrogen replacement therapy (ERT). When estrogen is used alone, it's called *unopposed estrogen therapy* because progestin isn't included to oppose the effects of the estrogen.

From the 1950s through the 1970s, doctors routinely prescribed *estrogen* (the female hormone responsible for giving you breasts, a curvy figure, a menstrual period, and more) by itself to treat menopausal symptoms. As the incidence of endometrial cancer in menopausal women climbed, researchers noticed that menopausal women were more prone to endometrial cancer if they were taking estrogen therapy. Researchers also found that if you take *progesterone* (the hormone that causes you to have a period and slough off the endometrial lining during your reproductive years) for a few days, the risk of endometrial cancer drops.

Here's why the addition of *progestin* (the synthetic form of progesterone) reduces the risk of endometrial cancer: Estrogen stimulates growth of the *endometrium* (uterine lining) to make a nice soft nest for a fertilized egg. Women were designed to shed the endometrial lining if the egg isn't fertilized. That way you clean out the nest each cycle to get ready for the next ovulation. Shedding the endometrium also serves another purpose because an occasional precancerous cell may be located among the endometrial lining. Stimulated growth month after month causes the occasional precancerous cell to multiply along with the normal cells. If you don't shed these precancerous cells, you're liable to develop endometrial cancer.

So researchers tried giving women *progestin* (the female hormone that causes changes in the uterus) for a few days. Just like in a natural cycle, when the progestin levels rise and then fall, the endometrial lining sheds — getting rid of any precancerous cells.

Menopausal women who don't take hormone therapy and women who are still menstruating (and shed their endometrial lining each month) rarely have problems with endometrial cancer.

Taking estrogen without balancing (or opposing) it with progestin is referred to as *unopposed estrogen therapy.* Women who've had a hysterectomy are really the only women who should receive estrogen alone. Without a uterus (which is removed during a hysterectomy), their chances of developing uterine cancer drop to zero. (Take a look at the "Unopposed estrogen therapy" section later in this chapter for more information.) For most other women, a combination of estrogen and progesterone is necessary.

Slaying the symptoms

For some women, perimenopausal symptoms are so severe that they truly interfere with their family lives, careers, self-esteem, or happiness.

Physicians have routinely prescribed hormone therapy to alleviate symptoms of perimenopause, such as hot flashes, vaginal dryness, disrupted sleep, mood swings, and so on, and it works fabulously. (Check out Chapter 2 for a full rundown of perimenopausal and menopausal symptoms.) Despite studies that suggest that there are health risks associated with hormone therapy, many women wouldn't want to go without hormone therapy because perimenopausal symptoms threaten their enjoyment of life.

People around the world have developed alternative therapies to alleviate the symptoms associated with perimenopause, and women in the Western world have started to choose alternatives to traditional hormone therapy. (Check out Chapter 5 for a rundown of alternative approaches.)

Preventing serious health problems with hormone therapy

Thanks to improvements in nutrition and healthcare, women living in the United States and Canada today may live into their 80s and 90s. Consider this: In 1900, North American women could expect to live to a ripe old age of 50 (barely into menopause). But today, the average lifespan is nearly 80 years (way beyond menopause). If you're an average woman (or better than average), you definitely want to consider shifting to a healthier lifestyle. And you may want to consider hormone therapy.

Here's why: Estrogen keeps the engine that is your body running smoothly, and you're going to be driving this car for quite some time (unlike the women in historical times who only drove the car while it was new). Think about how you maintain your car. It's one thing to be a quart low on oil when you're driving a couple miles to the grocery store — it may not do much damage. But taking a 2,000-mile trip when you're down a quart of oil is a completely different story. Your engine will burn up long before you reach the end of your journey. Just as you routinely check your oil level and add to it when necessary (before noticing a problem, we hope), you may need to intervene with medicine even when you're not sick to keep your body running smoothly.

The health problems standing in the way of staying active and comfortable are related to the fact that women produce lower levels of estrogen after becoming menopausal — which can be 20 or more years of your life. Low levels of estrogen can lead to health issues such as

✔ Osteoporosis

✔ Hardening of the arteries

✔ Heart disease (including heart attack and angina)

✔ Increased risk of some cancers

✔ Memory changes

Preventing some of these debilitating diseases and conditions is one of the reasons women elect to take hormone therapy. But most women first start hormone therapy to relieve the annoying symptoms of perimenopause, such as hot flashes, and continue to take it for years.

 Given the results of the recent Women's Health Initiative study and reassessments of other studies, hormone therapy seems to be only one leg of a four-legged stool. Hormone therapy provides greater benefit to women who also eat a healthy diet, get regular exercise, and visit their doctors regularly. We examine the benefits and risks of hormone therapy and the ramifications of long-term use in greater detail in Chapter 4.

Ticking through the Therapies

Every woman's body is different, and you can choose from a variety of regimens and many different types of hormones. We know that trying to get a handle on all the available hormones and therapies on the market can be overwhelming. So, in this section, the goal is to help you understand the different types of treatment programs women use and why they use them.

Estrogen plays such a large role in so many of your body's functions that compensating for the decreased production levels that menopause brings is a key component of most hormone therapies.

During menopause and beyond, the perimenopausal symptoms generally begin to subside, and the bigger concern is preventing, delaying, or treating health issues such as bone loss, cancer, and not-so-hot blood cholesterol levels.

Unopposed estrogen therapy

Unopposed estrogen therapy refers to a treatment program in which you receive only estrogen without any form of progesterone.

 Doctors only use unopposed estrogen if you have no uterus (you've had a hysterectomy) because taking estrogen without progestin can lead to endometrial cancer.

 If you have a history of blood-clotting problems (deep vein thrombosis), be careful about the types and doses of estrogen you use. In general, blood-clotting problems are associated with high dosages of estrogen — particularly with smokers. Today, physicians are trained to prescribe low-dosage estrogen. Whether or not you smoke, your physician generally starts you on the lowest dosage available and moves you to a higher dosage only if the lowest dosage doesn't relieve your problems. Low-dosage estrogen reduces your risk of blood clotting.

Some evidence shows that the estradiol form of estrogen is less likely to contribute to clotting problems than the conjugated types of estrogen. Because patches don't send estrogen to the liver where it stirs up trouble, they seem to be the delivery method of choice to avoid clotting problems.

 If you have an existing problem with liver or gallbladder disease, discuss these conditions with your doctor before using any type of estrogen. Patients with uncontrolled blood pressure shouldn't start on high doses of estrogen.

Treatment methods:

Your doctor will evaluate your symptoms and hormone levels in order to establish an appropriate dosage. You may take an estrogen pill every day or use a patch that you apply to your abdomen once or twice a week (the exact timing depends on the brand and your doctor's recommendations). Creams you apply to your skin (like you apply a moisturizer) are also available.

Benefits:

Taking unopposed estrogen boosts the amount of estrogen circulating in your bloodstream. This boost alleviates a variety of symptoms, including

- Anxiety
- Frequent urination
- Headaches
- Heart palpitations
- Hot flashes
- Interrupted sleep
- Memory lapses

✔ Mood swings and irritability

✔ Urinary incontinence

✔ Vaginal dryness and atrophy

Estrogen also has beneficial effects on bone maintenance, cholesterol levels, blood pressure, clotting factors, and the health of your blood vessels and heart tissue.

Taking unopposed estrogen also eliminates the premenstrual-symptom-like side effects of bloating, breast tenderness, and similar symptoms caused by progesterone.

Side effects:

If you take estrogen alone without progesterone or progestin, you won't have periods after menopause like you would with combination hormone therapy (see the "Combination therapy" section later in this chapter). Your *endometrium* (lining of your uterus) will continue to thicken and create quite a buildup. The buildup can lead to endometrial cancer (sometimes referred to as uterine cancer).

Other side effects from estrogen include breast fullness or tenderness, an increase in *triglycerides* (a type of fat in your blood), and an increase in blood pressure. These side effects can often be reduced or eliminated by decreasing the dosage or switching from the pill form of estrogen to an *estradiol* (active estrogen) patch that you place on your skin.

Sometimes side effects reflect a reaction to a dye or some inert (inactive) ingredient in an estrogen tablet and can be eliminated by switching from the pill to the patch. These side effects may include joint aches, muscle aches, skin irritation, and a burning sensation that accompanies urination.

Cautions:

Anyone who still has a uterus shouldn't use unopposed estrogen therapy because of the risk of endometrial cancer. If you have a history of breast cancer or you're experiencing undiagnosed vaginal bleeding, your physician won't prescribe unopposed estrogen therapy even if you've had a hysterectomy.

For women who have had a hysterectomy and have a family history of breast cancer, the answer isn't so clear. You and your doctor should have a frank discussion to decide if this type of therapy is for you.

You may have assumed this little pearl of wisdom, but we want to mention it anyway: Stay away from estrogen therapy if you're pregnant.

Combination therapy

Combination therapy means taking a combination of hormones as opposed to taking only estrogen. Generally, combination therapy consists of a combination of estrogen and progesterone (or the synthetic form of progesterone called _progestin_). Some women need to boost their _androgen_ (male hormone) levels as well, so testosterone or another male hormone may be part of the combination. Some women who experience a low libido take a small dose of testosterone in their "hormone cocktail."

Combining progesterone with estrogen provides the benefits of estrogen while reducing the risk of endometrial cancer that taking unopposed estrogen can heighten. The only bad part is that progestin/progesterone may slightly reduce some of the benefits of estrogen. The sole purpose for including progestin in hormone therapy is to reduce your risk of endometrial cancer.

If you have a uterus and you elect hormone therapy, your doctor will put you on some form of combination hormone therapy.

The combination products on the market contain varying doses of both estrogen and progesterone/progestin.

Treatment methods:

Combination therapy has a couple basic regimens for you and your medical advisor to choose from. If you're interested in hormone therapy and you don't have a medical history that rules it out, you and your doctor will review some information to decide what's right for you.

Combination hormone therapy comes in two basic forms:

✔ **Cyclic combination therapy:** With this form, you're taking estrogen and progestin in a cycle — generally the first part of the cycle involves estrogen; the second involves progestin. This combination will trigger a period because the progestin tells your uterus to shed the endometrial lining.

"But I thought menopause meant that you don't have a period," you say. Well you're right. You're not technically having a menstrual period; you're having vaginal bleeding. Drugs, not ovulation, trigger the periods that come with hormone therapy. Cyclic hormone therapy causes most women to have predictable vaginal bleeding, which can continue for years.

There are two common cyclic combination programs: In one regimen, you take estrogen every day of the month and estrogen and progestin together for the last 10 to 14 days of every cycle. In the other cyclic combination regimen, you take estrogen every day for 25 days of the month and progestin for 10 to 12 days. You take no medication for 3 to 6 days each month. You can expect to bleed when you're not taking the medication. Some people refer to this regimen as *sequential combination therapy* because you take the estrogen and progestin in a sequence.

✔ **Continuous combination therapy:** With this form of therapy, you take estrogen and progestin together every day. This approach seems to provide these benefits: lower risk of endometrial cancer, cessation of periods after six months or a year, and fewer progestin-related side effects in some women, especially bleeding.

Pills and patches on the market today combine the two hormones, making them easy to take. But some women who are sensitive to progestin experience fewer side effects when using a progestin cream and taking estrogen as a pill or patch. If you're bothered by side effects, talk with your doctor about experimenting with different dosages or forms to make you more comfortable.

Some women on combination therapy don't like the side effects they feel on the days they take progesterone. Don't stop taking progesterone/progestin without consulting your doctor, and take it for the exact length of time prescribed by your doctor. Taking just estrogen can lead to endometrial cancer. (For more information, see the "Unopposed estrogen therapy" section earlier in this chapter.)

Certain progestins are derived from testosterone and can help women who complain of low libido (sex drive) during and after menopause. The generic name for this progestin is *norethindrone.* Although norethindrone reduces many of the progestin side effects, it's not recommended for women with high LDL-cholesterol or tryglyceride levels. Like estrogen, you can take testosterone via creams, regular pills, pills you hold under your tongue, and vaginal suppositories. Doctors most commonly prescribe low-dosage skin creams and pills because these forms cause your body to absorb the testosterone more slowly, helping you avoid side effects caused by rapid shifts in your hormone levels.

Benefits:

Combination therapy should give you the best of all worlds — the benefits of estrogen (and perhaps testosterone) without the risks of endometrial cancer.

Continuous hormone therapy causes fewer side effects in women who are several years beyond menopause than in younger women. Plus, continuous hormone therapy causes fewer premenstrual-like symptoms than cyclic hormone therapy. If you're tired of tampons, keep in mind that one-third of women stop bleeding when they start the continuous combination therapy, many women stop monthly bleeding after two to three months, and most women stop monthly bleeding after one year of therapy. But proper dosages and delivery forms are needed to curb the side effects of progestin.

Women who have problems with their libido often find that a bit of testosterone in their hormone therapy gives it a boost.

Side effects:

Some women have a hard enough time tolerating human progesterone, and tolerating its synthetic cousin, progestin, is no easier. The progesterone/progestin can cause many premenstrual-syndrome-like symptoms, including

✔ Acne

✔ Bloating

✔ Depression

✔ Weight gain

Cautions:

Women with a history of breast cancer should not take hormone therapy, and those with a family history of breast cancer should carefully consider the risks. Also, women shouldn't take hormone therapy to prevent coronary artery disease or reduce the risk of heart attack, according to the recent results of the Women's Health Initiative study.

Women who have heart disease, uncontrolled diabetes, high blood pressure, high triglyceride levels, fibromyalgia, or depression aren't good candidates for continuous combination therapy because taking progestin every day often exacerbates these conditions.

Selective Estrogen Receptor Modulators (SERMs)

Meet the stealth bombers of the hormone therapy world. SERMs are manufactured designer drugs that target specific types of estrogen receptors (those areas that welcome and use estrogen) while blocking estrogen receptors in other parts of the body. SERMs don't contain estrogen. They stimulate estrogen receptors in the bone, brain, and cardiovascular system, but block the receptors in the breast and uterus.

This way, the drugs provide the benefits of estrogen to specific parts of the body without the drawbacks — the biggest drawback being the increased risk of breast cancer. The U.S. Food and Drug Administration (FDA) has approved two SERMS for use in the United States: tamoxifen and raloxifene.

Treatment methods:

Both tamoxifen and raloxifene are available in pill form and should be taken as directed by your physician.

Benefits:

SERMs may reduce bone loss in menopausal women, but not as well as estrogen. SERMs reduce the risk of breast cancer in women if taken for no more than five years. Unlike combination hormone therapy, SERMs have no negative effects on blood lipids, so they won't raise your triglyceride or LDL-cholesterol levels.

 A lot of research is still ongoing, and new types of SERMs are on their way. Targeting specific estrogen receptors for enrichment seems to be a very promising way to help women stay comfortable and healthy during and after menopause.

Side effects:

Unfortunately, SERM use brings some side effects:

- Insomnia
- Slight increased risk of endometrial cancer (with tamoxifen)
- Significant hot flashes

SERMs are beneficial to your blood cholesterol, but they do increase the risk of blood clots in your veins and lungs and may lead to strokes.

Cautions:

Anyone at risk of cardiovascular problems should
avoid SERMs. Also, women with hot flashes don't tol-
erate SERMs well, because SERMs tend to make the
symptoms worse.

Pills, Patches, and Pomades: A Smorgasbord of Delivery Options

Over the years, scientists have worked hard to provide hormone therapy that maximizes the benefits
and minimizes the side effects and inconveniences.
The result of all this effort is a smorgasbord of choices.
Basically, you have three paths to choose from to
deliver hormone therapy to your bloodstream: your
mouth (pill), skin (patch or cream), or vagina (cream,
gel, or ring). A fourth hormone-delivery path, muscle
(injection), exists but isn't used for hormone therapy.

The various delivery systems offer choices to suit the
personal and physiological preferences of a diverse
group of women. You and your doctor can experiment
to find the delivery methods and dosages that are
most effective for you.

Popping pills

Taking pills by mouth is a very traditional way of
ingesting medication, so understanding and correctly
performing the procedure is very easy. Getting the
exact dose that the doctor ordered is also simple
because the prescribed dosage is already loaded in
the pill; plus, the frequency is written on the label.
Hard to get this one wrong.

But, when you reach the age of 60 or 70, you may be
taking additional medications. For example, by that

time in their lives, many women are taking a multivitamin, extra calcium, high-blood-pressure medication, maybe something to strengthen their bones, and on and on. An additional pill in the parade can be a pain.

Pasting on a patch

Patches deliver drugs through the skin. In the old days (several years ago), bulky patches with a sometimes-skin-irritating reservoir of alcohol delivered the hormone. Today's patches are known as *matrix patches* because the hormone is actually incorporated in the adhesive that attaches to the skin. The patches currently on the market are much smaller, thinner, and less likely to irritate your skin than the patches of days gone by.

Patches have some advantages:

- ✔ You put them on once or twice a week.
- ✔ They deliver a constant supply of hormone so you have more consistent hormone levels in your blood.
- ✔ They're easier on your liver and digestive tract than pills are because they bypass these areas of your body and go straight into your bloodstream.

Really, the only problem you may have with a patch is that it could irritate your skin. Not many women have a problem with that though.

Applying creams

Vaginal lining responds very quickly to treatments applied directly to the area. Some women like vaginal creams because they deliver the hormones localized in a small area.

If you're treating vaginal dryness or atrophy yet worry about breast or endometrial cancer, a cream may be a good choice. For example, an estrogen cream relieves vaginal dryness and atrophy but doesn't increase your risk of breast cancer because the dosage is low and the estrogen stays put.

Creams are effective at treating your vagina, but they do nothing for your hot flashes, mood swings, bones, or blood cholesterol.

Cream applicators can be cumbersome to load and can make the whole process difficult and inexact. You may get more or less of a dose than you expected, and inevitably, you lose some cream from the vagina after the application. So you're never really sure exactly how much cream you've truly applied and how much you've lost. You may feel like putting a bit more in the applicator to compensate, but you don't know how much extra to add. Because applying creams is cumbersome, some women just quit doing it or don't apply the cream on a proper schedule.

New vaginal estrogen tablets have recently come on the market. These tablets are easy to apply, give a precise dose, and make less of a mess. One of these tablets is about the size of a baby aspirin, and you insert it high into the vagina with an applicator like you'd use for a tampon, only narrower. The pill dissolves slowly inside your body and releases small amounts of estrogen. You administer these pills about twice a week.

Slipping on a ring

This ring doesn't go on your finger; you place it in your vagina. Rings are fairly new in the United States, but women in Europe have been using them for quite a while.

The doctor usually inserts the flexible, hormone-containing ring initially; after that you can change it — usually every 90 days. The ring slowly delivers an even supply of hormones to your bloodstream. The dosage is very low, so it doesn't stimulate growth of the endometrial lining.

Don't worry: The ring is out of the way. But some women do have a problem tolerating the ring because they have short or narrow vaginas. Also, you can pop it out if you're straining on the toilet. But, if you're okay with a diaphragm, the ring isn't that much different.

A ring is a great option for women with vaginal and urinary tract symptoms, but it doesn't provide all the other health benefits of estrogen such as relief of perimenopausal symptoms and improved bone maintenance.

Searching for Sources

If you like to exchange recipes, here's a quick overview about how drug companies make these hormones. In the following sections, you can see that those folks in white lab coats have been very resourceful in finding ways to create hormones.

Estrogen

Some really clever scientists have found a variety of sources from which to make estrogen. Over the years, trying to get the right type and amount of estrogen into your body has been quite a challenge for the guys and gals in lab coats.

Before we get started with the recipes for hormone therapy, a quick reminder about the ins and outs of estrogen may be in order. Three types of estrogen exist: estrone, estradiol, and estriol. We mention this fact because all types of estrogen are not created equal. Here's a brief estrogen primer:

- ✔ **Estradiol** is the biologically active type of estrogen and the most potent form of human estrogen. It's a player in hundreds of bodily functions.

- ✔ **Estrone** isn't the workhorse that estradiol is; estrone is more like the warehouse variety of estrogen that's stored in your body fat. It can be turned into estradiol, but only in pre-menopausal ovaries.

- ✔ As for **estriol,** fuggetaboutit — in this context anyway. Estriol is mostly found in pregnant women.

All right. Now that that's taken care of, here are the sources of estrogen that scientists have come up with:

- ✔ Conjugated equine estrogen
- ✔ Estradiol estrogen
- ✔ Esterified estrogen
- ✔ Estropipate
- ✔ Micronized estradiol

Progestin

Most of the side effects attributed to hormone therapy are the result of the progestin, but progestin protects you from developing endometrial cancer. Because every woman's body is different, you may need to do some experimenting to figure out which progestin is right for you.

Adding progestin to the hormone therapy mix does seem to reduce the benefits estrogen can have on

your cholesterol levels and increase changes to
your mood.

There are three types of progestin on the market:

- ✔ Progesterone
- ✔ Medroxyprogesterone acetate (MPA)
- ✔ Progestin derived from testosterone

Combinations of estrogen and progestin

For convenience's sake, you may want to combine
estrogen and progestin into a single pill or patch.

A couple brands on the market contain conjugated
estrogen with a progestin called medroxyprogesterone acetate (MPA). The U.S. Food and Drug
Administration approved MPA for women having trouble with their periods. MPA helps prevent the
endometrium (uterine lining) from thickening too
much and helps regulate periods. MPA is useful in
combination hormone therapy because it inhibits the
over-thickening of your endometrium, so it lowers
your risk of endometrial cancer.

Conjugated estrogen and MPA is a commonly prescribed combination therapy and can be administered as either sequential courses of estrogen
followed by progestin or as continuous combination
therapy (see the "Combination therapy" section earlier in this chapter).

Today, new combination therapies use a progestin
derived from testosterone, *norethindrone acetate,*
instead of MPA because it causes less vaginal bleeding. You can get a combination therapy in both patch
and pill forms. The combination patch administers

the estradiol form of estrogen and norethindrone acetate. Many women like the patch because you don't have to remember to take a pill and it's convenient to have both hormones delivered in a single patch.

Androgens

When we talk about *androgens* (male hormones), we're mainly talking about testosterone.

You may need to include androgens (most likely testosterone) in your hormone therapy for a couple of reasons. If you've become menopausal due to surgery (removal of your ovaries), your androgens may take a nosedive very quickly. You may want to bump up your androgens because they help bone maintenance and libido. Women who experience natural menopause may need androgens in the regimen because estrogen supplements may decrease the amount of physiologically active testosterone in your bloodstream (which could lower your libido and lessen muscle tone).

Using too high a dose of testosterone has some side effects: acne, oily skin, hair loss, unwanted hair, and a deeper voice. Rest assured that prescribed dosages are rarely high enough to trigger these side effects.

Doing the Dosing

The guideline that every doctor uses is this: Use the smallest dose possible to alleviate symptoms and health risks while minimizing the side effects. That said, women react to hormone supplements very differently. No one knows why a particular regimen causes one woman to experience side effects and another to sing its praises from the rooftop.

Your doc will review your personal medical history,
your family medical history, and the results of your
physical examination and lab work. He'll also want to
consider what conditions or problems you're trying
to overcome or prevent. (For example: Are we talking
about lessening perimenopausal symptoms or preventing osteoporosis after menopause?) Share your
personal preferences and prejudices with your doctor
at this time as well. (Do you have a hard time swal-
lowing pills? Do you forget to take medicine? Are you
determined to throw away the tampons as soon as
possible? These kinds of issues are the ones you'll
want to talk about.)

During perimenopause, some women experience
symptoms that make life absolutely miserable.
Doctors may try prescribing a hormone therapy regimen in these cases. Here are the standard schedules
for hormone therapy:

- ✔ **Cyclic:** Take estrogen daily and add progestin
  for 10 to 14 days per month.

- ✔ **Cyclic/Sequential:** Take estrogen for 25 days
  each month and progestin for 10 to 12 days each
  month. No medication is used for 3 to 6 days
  per month. Vaginal bleeding is expected during
  the period when no medication is taken.

- ✔ **Continuous:** Take estrogen and progestin daily.
  You generally have no vaginal bleeding after a
  few months of using continuous hormone
  therapy (which is why many women like this
  regimen).

- ✔ **Patch:** Apply a *transdermal* (skin) patch twice a
  week (or as directed) to an area of the body not
  exposed directly to the sun.

If you have issues with your libido, your doctor takes
it into the equation when prescribing hormone
therapy. Convenience is also an issue. Convenience

considerations include how many other medications you take (do you really want to take more pills or use a patch), the cost, and how anxious you are to quit bleeding every month. As far as the last issue goes, *sequential/cyclical therapy* (taking estrogen for part of the month and progestin another part of the month) results in continuing your periods for some time, but *continuous combination therapy* (taking both estrogen and progestin at the same time every day) generally stops your periods. SERMs also eliminate your periods.

Your doctor may need to do some experimenting with different products to find the right one for you — one that will eliminate your symptoms while producing the fewest side effects.

Most doctors start out using standard doses but then customize dosages to the individual. With hormone therapy, one size doesn't fit all. So your doctor may take a number of blood samples to figure out where your hormones are and try to administer dosages that will get your hormones to an appropriate target level.

It's not the estrogen!

Many reports and books make a huge deal about the fact that no scientific evidence links changes in estrogen levels to a declining libido. These publications then make the leap to erroneously conclude that hormones have nothing to do with libido. Although the estrogen, itself, may not play the deciding role in libido regulation, the *balance* between estrogen and testosterone likely makes a difference.

This subject is a bit controversial so we want to give you both sides of the argument. On one side are scientists who conclude that supplementing your testosterone during menopause increases your libido. On the other side are the lab coats who believe that the science doesn't exist to show that prescribing testosterone is either safe or effective for women who complain of low libido.

Testosterone is produced naturally by women's ovaries and has a very positive impact on your libido, mood, vitality, sense of well-being, bone, and muscle. But, even before menopause, your body slows down its production of testosterone. After menopause, you produce about half as much testosterone as you produced during your reproductive years. So it's not unusual for your libido to decline if your testosterone levels are too low.

You don't want to have too much testosterone either — it can promote breast and liver cancer. Plus, too much testosterone relative to estrogen can unleash the effects of testosterone that estrogen had been keeping under control, such as facial hair, increased libido, redistribution of body fat (it moves to the middle of your body), and acne.

Some doctors shy away from prescribing testosterone as part of hormone therapy (HT) because they're afraid of upsetting the estrogen/testosterone balance and causing unpleasant side effects. The trick, whether you're taking HT with testosterone or not, is to keep testosterone levels high enough to avoid one set of side effects (including low libido) and in balance with the other hormones to avoid another set of side effects (facial hair or acne, for example).

Those folks in the scientific and medical communities who view testosterone as a worthy treatment for libido problems believe that the bad side effects felt by some women are caused by excessively high dosages of testosterone. Proponents of testosterone use suggest using very low dosages and maintaining a balance between the levels of testosterone and estrogen.

Chapter 4

Making the Decision about Hormone Therapy

● ●

In This Chapter

▶ Recognizing a variety of opinions

▶ Connecting the studies to the headlines

▶ Weighing your options during perimenopause

▶ Weighing your options during menopause

● ●

*W*e want to start this chapter by encouraging you to return to it periodically over the next few years. Your decisions about coping with peri-menopause and menopause will probably change as your health changes, your priorities shift, and new options become available. This evaluation process doesn't end with a one-time pronouncement that you have to follow for the rest of your life. You can (and should!) revisit your alternatives periodically.

Outlining Attitudes about HT

Most women going through the change fall into one of three camps when it comes to hormone therapy (HT).

✔ "Natural is beautiful. If we were meant to have estrogen all our lives, we would have been born that way."

✔ "There's no way I want to live a day without my hormones!"

✔ "I've tried hormones, and they were awful. I guess I'll just have to put up with the symptoms."

Over time, you may move from one camp to the next — and then back again. If your symptoms interfere with the quality of your life during perimenopause, you may want to take hormones for a few years to ease the transition into menopause and then taper off medication as your symptoms decrease.

The purpose of HT is to bring your hormones into a "healthy" balance. The "natural is beautiful" group argues that what's normal at 25 isn't normal at 55, and they're correct. Unfortunately, the low levels of estrogen that are "normal" at 55 often result in physical and mental discomfort.

The problem is that your body doesn't produce a substitute for estrogen when your ovaries quit producing the hormone. When your body stops getting the estrogen it's used to having, it lets you know with messages in the form of hot flashes, memory lapses, vaginal dryness, bone loss, and shifting blood cholesterol levels, all of which are typical of sustained, low levels of estrogen.

Updating HT recommendations

The results from the Women's Health Initiative (WHI) study released in 2002 seemed to put the kibosh on hormone therapy (HT). The study evaluated the use of a combination estrogen and progestin as a means of lowering the risk of cardiovascular disease in women. After several years, the answer became clear. Not only did this combination of hormones *not* lower the risk of cardiovascular disease, it actually increased the risk of breast cancer, heart attacks, strokes, and blood clots. Based on these findings, the National Institutes of Health, the sponsor of the study, terminated the trial several years ahead of schedule.

But the WHI findings are neither surprising nor applicable to all forms of HT. The study evaluated the use of a specific HT product (conjugated equine estrogen plus MPA progestin). This specific estrogen product, derived from female horse urine, is one of the most commonly prescribed forms, but one that was already known to have problems. Other major studies performed in the 1980s and 1990s showed that horse-derived estrogens may produce higher risks of heart disease than the natural estradiol form of estrogen.

The specific HT product administered in the test uses MPA (medroxyprogesterone acetate) as the progestin part of the therapy; this also wasn't the best choice. Researchers have known for more than ten years that MPA causes more blood vessel damage and reverses more of the positive effects of estrogen than natural progesterone.

In essence, the WHI study simply confirms the information that we've known for about 20 years — the most-prescribed HT product is not a good choice for menopausal women.

To be fair, the WHI study is one of the biggest, best organized, and best controlled studies of HT and its effects on women's health ever conducted. If you want to know how conjugated estrogen and MPA affect women after menopause, the WHI has some hard facts on the benefits and risks. But, the study leads us to wonder if *all* HT regimens would have the same results. We know that pills have different effects than patches, and we know that conjugated estrogen has different effects than estradiol estrogen. We don't know whether these other HT regimens have the same health risks as the one tested in the WHI study.

If you have a family or personal history that includes osteoporosis or colorectal cancer, HT may be the right choice for you. Keep in mind that other medications can be helpful too. (Check out Chapter 6 for information on treating osteoporosis without hormones.)

Taking hormone therapy does present health risks. Estrogen encourages the growth of some breast cancers and may also be a problem for women with gallbladder or liver problems, blood clots, or undiagnosed vaginal bleeding. So how do you decide? Businesspeople often perform cost-benefit analyses, a very rational approach in which you list the benefits and the costs (in this case risks) and make a logical decision. The information in this chapter (and throughout this book) can help you perform a cost-benefit analysis.

As with any personal decision, you also have to consider your values, lifestyle preferences, and personal prejudices and preferences — illogical as some of them may be. Also, look at your medical history and that of your family. You may eventually face the same medical problems that affect your parents, siblings, or grandparents. We help you sort through these issues, too.

Realizing the Benefits of HT

HT relieves perimenopausal and menopausal symptoms and protects your body against a variety of serious medical conditions. You can find information about these benefits throughout this book (Chapter 3 is a good place to start), but we put them all together here so you can do a quick side-by-side comparison as you're trying to make your decision.

HT relieves

- ✔ Bone deterioration
- ✔ Fuzzy thinking
- ✔ Hot flashes
- ✔ Insomnia and fitful sleep due to hot flashes or night sweats
- ✔ Memory lapses
- ✔ Vaginal dryness and *vaginal atrophy* (thinning and shrinking)

Some evidence points to the fact that the mental and emotional symptoms are actually worse during peri-menopause than after you're officially menopausal. The wild hormone fluctuations are probably the culprit.

REMEMBER

If you're experiencing many of the peri-menopausal symptoms described in the "Figuring out just how bad it really is" sidebar in this chapter, but they appear at about the same time each month — prior to your period — and then go away for some length of time during each menstrual cycle, you probably have pre-menstrual syndrome rather than peri-menopausal symptoms.

By raising the level of estrogen in your body during the latter 20 to 40 years of your life, you can protect yourself against a number of disabling conditions:

- ✔ Cardiovascular disease, which includes arteriosclerosis, heart attack, and heart disease
- ✔ Colon cancer
- ✔ Elevated LDL ("bad" cholesterol) and *triglyceride* (another bad cholesterol) levels
- ✔ Osteoporosis (weakening of the bones)

Figuring out just how bad it really is

This little quiz is designed to help you decide whether you're experiencing perimenopausal symptoms, and if so, whether they're interfering with your quality of life. The responses are ranked in order from least debilitating to most. The more debilitating, the greater the chance that these symptoms are interfering with your life. There are no cut-off points and no target scores — you be the judge.

How often do you experience hot flashes or night sweats?

- ✔ Never.
- ✔ Several times a week, but I can deal with it.
- ✔ Several times a day, and they interfere with my activities.
- ✔ So often that I'm going nuts.

How often do you experience interrupted sleep or insomnia?

- ✔ About the same as I have in the past.
- ✔ Once in a while, but I simply don't sleep as well as I used to.
- ✔ I wake up a couple times a night, and I have a hard time getting back to sleep.
- ✔ I feel like a zombie because I'm awake so much of the night.

Do you feel irritable, anxious, or apprehensive?

- ✔ No more than usual.
- ✔ I'm more irritable, anxious, or apprehensive than I used to be.
- ✔ I sometimes cry at the drop of a hat, and other times, I just want to be alone.
- ✔ I'm driving my family and coworkers nuts because I fly into a rage one minute and I'm fine the next.

Are you experiencing vaginal dryness, burning, or itching?

✓ No more than usual.

✓ Intercourse is uncomfortable at times.

✓ My partner and I have cut down on intercourse because it's painful, and I still feel itchy and uncomfortable.

✓ My vagina feels uncomfortable and itchy when doing everyday activities.

Do you experience any other perimenopausal problems? (Circle all that apply.)

✓ I experience perimenopausal-like symptoms prior to my period, but then they go away.

✓ I've noticed my headaches are getting more frequent.

✓ My skin feels prickly, like bugs are crawling on me.

✓ I leak urine when I laugh, exercise, or sneeze.

✓ I seem to leak urine no matter what type of activity I'm doing.

✓ I have frequent memory lapses and have a hard time concentrating.

✓ My heartbeat flutters or pounds rapidly, sometimes when I'm just sitting or resting.

If you experience many of these symptoms but they appear at about the same time each month — prior to your period — and then go away for some length of time during each menstrual cycle, you probably have premenstrual syndrome rather than perimenopausal symptoms.

You may be the type of woman who marches through perimenopause, refusing to let those annoying symptoms interfere with your life. Maybe getting relief from the symptoms just didn't seem to be worth the risks that HT may contribute to other health problems. Or maybe you barely experienced any symptoms.

As you approach menopause, the risks and rewards of HT may look different to you. The statistics, which we put on paper in the following sections, are fairly dramatic. The decision scales may become more balanced; you may even throw up your hands and say, "Damned if I do, damned if I don't." What can you do to sort through the decision-making process? Read on. While you're reading, take your family medical history and personal health concerns into account. And keep in mind that you can always take a fresh look at the situation next month or next year.

Helping your heart stay healthy

Out of a group of 100 women who are 50 years old, 20 of them will develop heart disease before their 80th birthday. But, if you put all 100 women on hormones, only 10 will develop heart disease before they turn 80. (Figure 4-1 provides a graphic representation.)

Pretty impressive, but here's the caveat: During the first and second years of hormone use, the risk of heart disease is actually greater than it is without hormones. After the second year, researchers are divided on the benefits of hormone therapy. A very large and frequently mentioned study, the Nurses' Health Study, found the risk of heart disease decreases after the second year of hormone use, and over time, the use of estrogen cuts the risk of heart disease in half.

The Nurses' Health Study isn't the only study that showed women using hormone therapy had a lower risk of heart disease. So, many people were surprised when the Women's Health Initiative (WHI) study recently concluded that hormone therapy actually increases the risk of heart disease with extended use. Why did the WHI findings differ so radically from prior studies? Did the specific type of combination therapy (Prempro) the WHI participants used cause the results? The medical community hasn't formulated an answer to those questions quite yet, but researchers are fast at work to see if other types of hormones yield the same result.

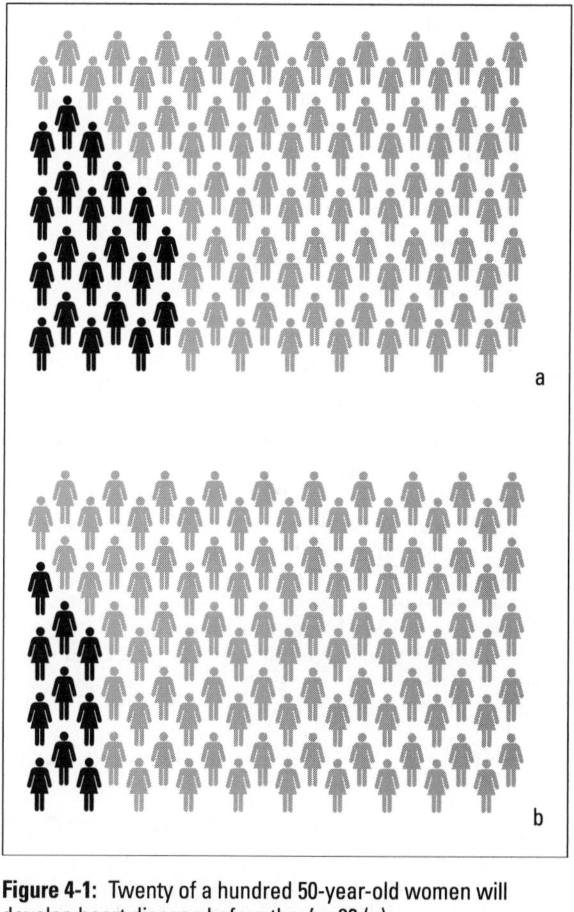

Figure 4-1: Twenty of a hundred 50-year-old women will develop heart disease before they're 80 (a).
If they all take HT, that number is cut in half (b).

The WHI results have already caused two women doctors to head back to the books to reevaluate the old studies. What did they find during their reexamination? A group of women with similar lifestyles (they exercise, they don't drink a lot of alcohol, and they eat a healthy diet) had less heart disease than other women whether or not they took hormones.

At this point in time, it appears that hormone therapy shouldn't be the first line of defense in treating or preventing heart disease or heart attack. And you should avoid hormone therapy if you have a history of heart disease or heart attack. The first line of defense against heart disease and heart attack should be a healthy diet, regular exercise, and an overall healthy lifestyle.

It's important to note that researchers stopped the WHI study, but they didn't put the breaks on because participants were in grave danger of dying from a heart attack or heart disease. (Although use of hormone therapy seemed to increase the risk of heart attack, it didn't increase the risk of *dying* from a heart attack.) Researchers halted the study because of the increased risk in breast cancer.

What about other types of cardiovascular disease such as fatty blood (high LDL and triglyceride levels) and *hypertension* (high blood pressure)? Glad you asked. Estrogen is a mixed bag as far as cholesterol and triglycerides are concerned:

- Estrogen lowers LDL levels (by as much as 15 percent in one study).

- Some forms of estrogen raise HDL ("good" cholesterol) levels.

- Oral estrogen seems to increase triglycerides (boo!), but the patch tends to lower triglycerides (yeah!).

The moral of this story is that if you have a problem with blood cholesterol and triglycerides, you need to find the right type of estrogen to keep them in check.

 Estrogen's benefits are clearer in relation to high blood pressure. It helps dilate blood vessels and improve blood flow, both of which lower your blood pressure.

The jury is still out on the impact of estrogen on stroke. High doses of estrogen seem to increase the risk of stroke slightly in menopausal women. This shouldn't be a problem anymore because today's HT regimens use low-dosage estrogen. Still, research confirms a slight increase in the risk of stroke during the first two years of use. After the first two years, estrogen actually seems to lower the risk of stroke in women taking HT.

Lifting the veil on combination HT and your heart

Now, when you add *progestin* (synthetic forms of the hormone progesterone) to the hormone therapy, everything changes. Progestins seem to dull the positive effects of estrogen on your cardiovascular system. Here are the findings for HT containing estrogen and progestin:

- ✔ It lowers HDL cholesterol (when taken in pill form).
- ✔ It raises triglycerides (when taken in pill form).

Unfortunately, if you have a uterus and want to take HT, the progestin must be included. But a variety of progestins are available, and patches have less of a negative impact on cholesterol than pills. Natural progesterone, ground up so your body can absorb it, doesn't seem to dull the effects of estrogen as much as progestins.

Before the WHI study, most doctors agreed that women could lower their risk of cardiovascular problems by using HT. Most doctors now agree that combination HT shouldn't be the first line of defense against cardiovascular disease.

Here's the $64-million question: Could it be that conjugated estrogen and MPA progestin (the hormone therapy tested in the WHI study) produce more hazardous side effects than other, more natural forms of hormone therapy (estradiol and natural progesterone, for example)? Well, we all have to stay tuned for the answer to that question.

It's not really appropriate to take the results of the WHI study and say that all combination hormone therapy regimens would create the same hazards to your cardiovascular system. But just so you know, here's what the WHI study concluded regarding the Prempro combination HT regimen:

✔ The risk of stroke doesn't increase during the first year of HT use, but it increases over time — after the first year for about five years (even in healthy women).

✔ Your risk of suffering a heart attack increases while taking HT, *but* you're not more likely to die of a heart attack while taking HT compared to women who don't take HT at all.

Avoiding bone breaks

HT dramatically reduces the risk of osteoporosis and the debilitating results of the disease in Caucasian and Asian women (check out Figure 4-2). The top figure (a) shows the number of women out of 100 who will suffer a hip fracture after age 50 — 15. The bottom figure (b) shows the number of hip fractures in women 50 or older who take hormone therapy — 11.

Because African American women have a lower incidence of osteoporosis, use of HT only slightly lowers their risk of fracture.

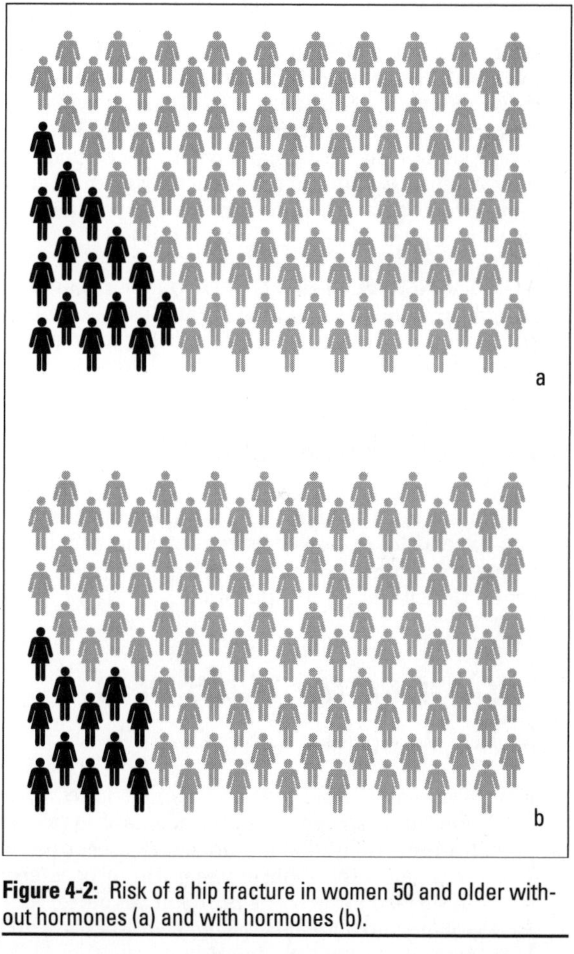

Figure 4-2: Risk of a hip fracture in women 50 and older without hormones (a) and with hormones (b).

Most women lose about 3 percent of bone mass each year after menopause. Postmenopausal women who take HT regularly for ten years don't lose bone mass; they actually increase their bone mass by about 6 percent!

Because women on HT regimens lose less bone (or even build bone) during menopause, they also have a lower incidence of hip fractures. HT users are about 25 percent less likely to fracture a hip. That stat is pretty significant, particularly when you consider how debilitating hip fractures are to women after menopause. (Many women require care for the rest of their lives after suffering a broken hip.)

The protective effects of HT on your bones only last as long as you take hormones. So when you stop — wham! — you begin losing bone mass quickly.

Keeping colon cancer at bay

Here's another one of those "we don't know exactly why, but it does" benefits of HT. While you take HT, you have a slightly lower risk of developing colon cancer. After you discontinue using hormones, the protection gradually disappears.

Considering the Risks of HT

HT also presents some risks to women:

- ✔ **It increases your risk of endometrial cancer if you take estrogen without also taking progesterone.** Today, doctors no longer prescribe estrogen without balancing it with progesterone, so this isn't much of a problem anymore. Unless you've had a hysterectomy, your doctor won't prescribe estrogen alone.

above pre menop ~

✔ **It increases your risk of gallbladder problems.**
Although we have the statistics to prove that HT
increases your risk of gallstones (particularly
when taken in pill form for more than five
years), researchers don't know the particulars
concerning why this is the case. The risk can be
lowered by using a patch instead of a pill.

✔ **It may increase your risk of breast cancer.**
Some breast cancers, but not all breast cancers,
depend on estrogen to grow. Because HT raises
estrogen levels, taking it may encourage estro-
gen-related breast cancer. The evidence is stack-
ing up on this issue.

✔ **It may increase your risk of deep-vein blood
clots.** If you experienced clotting during a pregnancy or while using birth-control pills, you may
have a problem with HT as well, particularly if
you smoke.

✔ **It may increase your risk of heart attack and
coronary heart disease.** The scales are starting
to tip in the direction that HT may actually
increase your risk of heart problems rather than
lower it — the jury is still out. This finding may
be less true of HT that uses skin patches as the
method of delivery and estradiol as the estrogen, as opposed to other forms of HT.

Having trouble deciding if you're at risk for osteoporosis, cardiovascular disease, or breast cancer? We
have three little quizzes to help you look objectively
at your risk factors in Figures 4-3, 4-4, and 4-5. The lists
are a very simple first step to assess your risks —
high, low, or in between. You can't predict your
chances of getting a particular disease based on your
answers, but the more statements you agree with, the
greater your risk for that condition.

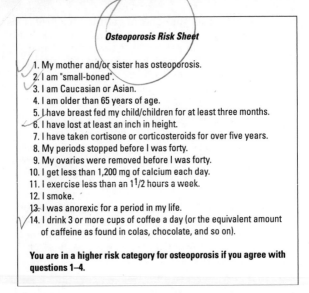

Osteoporosis Risk Sheet

1. My mother and/or sister has osteoporosis.
2. I am "small-boned".
3. I am Caucasian or Asian.
4. I am older than 65 years of age.
5. I have breast fed my child/children for at least three months.
6. I have lost at least an inch in height.
7. I have taken cortisone or corticosteroids for over five years.
8. My periods stopped before I was forty.
9. My ovaries were removed before I was forty.
10. I get less than 1,200 mg of calcium each day.
11. I exercise less than an 1 1/2 hours a week.
12. I smoke.
13. I was anorexic for a period in my life.
14. I drink 3 or more cups of coffee a day (or the equivalent amount of caffeine as found in colas, chocolate, and so on).

You are in a higher risk category for osteoporosis if you agree with questions 1–4.

Figure 4-3: Evaluating your risk for osteoporosis.

It's important to realize that *risk* is not the same as *certainty*. We all know people who smoked and drank and lived a long life and others who lived healthy and exercised and died of a heart attack well before their time. But, in between these unlikely extremes, you can evaluate your risk factors and try to take some steps to improve your chances of preventing disease.

Many women choose to weigh their risk of osteoporosis and cardiovascular disease against their risk of breast cancer because HT protects you from osteoporosis but may raise your risk for breast cancer, and depending on what form of HT you take, it may or may not help protect you from heart disease.

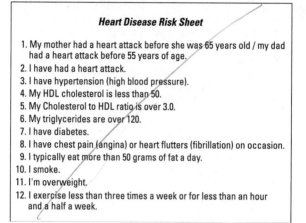

Figure 4-4: Evaluating your risk for heart disease.

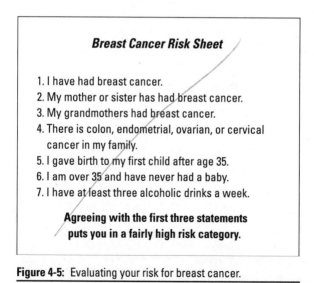

Figure 4-5: Evaluating your risk for breast cancer.

If you're at great risk of osteoporosis or cardiovascular disease but have few risk factors for breast cancer, HT may be for you. If you're at great risk for breast cancer, you may want to consider other alternatives for protecting your bones and heart. Chapters 5 and 6 give you some great ideas about alternatives.

Some of the risk factors for each of the conditions are things that you can control by modifying your lifestyle, eating preferences, or other behaviors. You can lower these risks immediately by making some changes.

Some studies indicate that use of HT slightly increases your risk of breast cancer (other studies show no effect whatsoever — so it's still controversial). If you're worried about your risk of breast cancer, take an objective look at your personal risk factors for the disease.

Summing Up the Studies

If you've made it this far through the chapter, you've digested a lot of information, and your plate is probably still full. We thought we'd included a little synopsis at this point to help you separate your peas from your potatoes, regroup, re-energize, and re-weigh the risks and benefits associated with hormone therapy.

You should realize that the best-studied type of HT is the regimen in which women take a daily pill that contains both conjugated equine estrogen and MPA progestin. Studies of other regimens are more scattered in terms of the size of the study group and the types of HT investigated. So these results are heavily biased toward the benefits and risks of combination therapy using conjugated estrogen and MPA progestin. (For more information on all the different types of therapies and hormones, check out Chapter 3.) Tables 4-1 and 4-2 provide a summary of the short- and long-term benefits and risks of HT.

Table 4-1	Just the Facts Ma'am: HT Benefits during Use	
Short-Term Use (Less Than Five Years)	**Long-Term Use (Five Years or More)**
Improved mental skills (verbal memory and reasoning)	Increased bone density
Improved sense of well-being	Reduction of hip fractures
Decrease in sleep interruption	Reduction of spinal fractures
Decrease in *urogenital atrophy* (atrophy of the vagina and urinary tract)	Reduction of colon cancer
Decrease in mood swings	Decrease in dementia
Decrease in hot flashes	

Table 4-2	Just the Facts Ma'am, Part II: HT Risks during Use	
Short-Term Use (Less Than Five Years)	**Long Term Use (Five Years or More)**
Possible increase in breast cancer	Increase in breast cancer
Increase in gallbladder disease	Significant increase in gallbladder disease

(continued)

Table 4-2 *(continued)*	
Short-Term Use (Less Than Five Years)	*Long Term Use (Five Years or More)*
Increase in heart attack	Slight increase in heart attack
Slight increase in stroke	Slight increase in stroke
Significant increase in deep-vein clots	Increase in deep-vein clots

Presenting the Options for Perimenopause

In the following sections, we present several ways that women deal with perimenopausal symptoms. Even though we group them into individual options, you may want to mix and match. For example, we discuss diet and exercise, herbal solutions, and HT in separate sections. But adopting better eating and exercise habits can only enhance the positive aspects of herbs or HT.

Option 1: The lifestyle solution

If you're perimenopausal and your symptoms annoy you but rarely interfere with your life, you may want to make some lifestyle changes to alleviate them. Many women find that some of the symptoms of perimenopause fade with a renewed focus on getting or staying fit.

Some of the anxiety and irritability you're experiencing probably stems from feeling out of control about the changes going on with your body. Adding a couple pounds a year and losing muscle tone isn't unusual for perimenopausal women, but it's also not caused by changes in your hormones. As people move into their 40s and 50s, they often devote less time to their personal needs than they devote to the demands of their families and careers. A healthy diet and exercise plan can put you in control of your body and improve your state of mind.

Regular physical activity improves mental functions such as memory, concentration, self-confidence, and self-esteem. It also reduces stress, which can trigger hot flashes, interrupted sleep, and irritability. But it's not all mental. Only about 1 in 20 women who exercise regularly report experiencing hot flashes, compared to 1 out of 4 less-active women.

Eating a healthy diet will boost your immune system, help maintain bone density, and keep your blood lean so you lower your risk of cardiovascular disease and reverse some of the effects of low estrogen levels that define menopause.

Incorporating soy into your diet helps lower your cholesterol, boost your immune system, and prevent hot flashes, and it may lower your risk of breast cancer. (Check out Chapter 5 for more on soy.)

Option 2: The herbal solution

For most women, perimenopausal symptoms are not life threatening so using drugs and hormones to relieve symptoms may seem like using a shotgun to kill mosquitoes.

You may want to consider some non-HT alternatives to alleviate your symptoms. These alternatives can be as diverse as herbs, relaxation techniques, and vaginal lubricants. Herbs of interest for relieving perimenopausal symptoms include black cohosh, soy, dong quai, and ginseng. We cover herbal solutions in detail in Chapter 5.

Stress often triggers hot flashes and anxiety or irritability, so now is a great time to practice relaxation techniques regularly. Don't worry: You don't need to go to Nepal to find a guru. Just take a few minutes each day to do an activity you enjoy, practice some breathing techniques, and give someone a hug. *Biofeedback techniques* (psychological therapy in which you use your mind to control certain body functions) can help you take charge of your breathing and heart rate and lessen your reactions to stressful events or situations.

Find out what works for you to reduce the stress in your life — maybe it's yoga, walking, music, or a weekly massage. Chapter 5 explores alternative options.

Option 3: The HT solution

Maybe you aren't wild about taking medication, but your symptoms are interfering with your quality of life; HT may be the answer. HT has been shown to relieve hot flashes because estrogen helps regulate body temperature. In addition, estrogen improves sleep and lowers anxiety by increasing the production and extending the action of *serotonin* (a brain chemical that regulates moods and activity level). Serotonin boosts concentration, improves pain tolerance, enhances memory, and regulates adrenaline so you avoid heart palpitations. Progesterone has been added to the HT regimen to reduce the risk of endometrial cancer that estrogen-only HT would present.

Many women choose to take HT to get rid of their annoying perimenopausal symptoms and may get added protection for their bones and hearts.

 If you decide that HT is for you, you still have the option of not using the therapy later on. After a few years, perimenopausal symptoms subside (they don't last forever), and you may decide to limit your use of HT to perimenopause.

The HT option is almost required for women who have their ovaries removed before menopause. Often HT is prescribed prior to surgery or immediately thereafter. Removal of your ovaries is quite a shock to your body because hormone production abruptly ceases. HT can help absorb the shock by replacing the hormones and smoothing things over so you don't experience intense menopausal symptoms, bone loss, or changes in your blood cholesterol.

 Many types of estrogen and progesterone are available in many different combinations. Some combinations may make you feel worse; others may make you feel better. If you're feeling worse, don't simply continue with the regimen or just give up — go back to your doctor and discuss the situation.

 While you're working the kinks out of your HT program, monitor your symptoms and any adverse reactions and write them down. Having some notes when you visit your doctor can help make the meeting more productive. You can accurately describe the symptoms and reactions to your doctor, and the two of you can come up with a treatment plan that works for you.

It may take your doctor time and you may have to try a couple of different formulas to find the correct therapy for you. Remember the lesson of the hospital gown: One size fits no one. If you're not comfortable with your doctor, find a medical advisor with whom you can work.

Finding Your Comfort Zone

This chapter takes a look at risk factors for various medical conditions that are associated with estrogen or the lack of it. But you can't make a decision about HT without considering your lifestyle and your personal preferences.

Some women are frightened at the thought of taking another medication; others fear having a heart attack. Some women make a concerted effort to improve their health by committing to more exercise and a healthier diet; others are dedicated couch potatoes. Some women live in families who support new endeavors; others live in families who ridicule change.

The following sections help you assess some of these touchy-feely personal values to see if you're likely to protect your health more successfully using diet, exercise, and non-HT alternatives or whether HT presents you with the best chances for success. Consider these factors as a piece of your HT decision-making puzzle.

Signs that HT is not for you

To get an HT program working for you, you have to communicate well with your doctor and share a sense of trust with him or her. If you aren't in that frame of mind, you may not have success with an HT program.

And, if you're the type of woman who is wary of
traditional medicine, pharmaceuticals, synthetic
drugs, or all of the above, you may want try some of
the alternatives to HT. You can always reevaluate your
condition and your comfort zone in the future.

 Read the following statements and see if you
agree with them. If you're in agreement with a
lot of these statements, you may want to try HT
alternatives including a healthy diet, exercise,
herbal alternatives, and other preventative
treatments.

✔ I have had breast cancer.

✔ My mother, sister, or daughter has had breast
cancer.

✔ I have coronary heart disease.

✔ I don't have or can live with my hot flashes,
interrupted sleep, or other symptoms caused by
hormonal changes.

✔ I have a history of unexplained blood clots,
deep-vein thrombosis, or blood clots in my
lungs *(pulmonary embolism)*.

✔ I don't like taking medication and believe herbs
can do a better job than drugs.

✔ I typically eat a healthy diet that includes at
least five servings of fruits and vegetables a day.

✔ I exercise regularly, and I'm successful at maintaining my target weight.

✔ I think physicians and pharmaceutical companies are just out to make money from women
going through menopause.

✔ I haven't gone to a doctor in years and don't
plan on starting now.

✔ My mother said she never had any problems going through menopause without hormones, and I don't think I will either.

✔ I have very few risk factors for osteoporosis or cardiovascular disease.

Signs that you're a good candidate for HT

No one wants to take medicine just to take it. Women who take HT during menopause are concerned about preventing disease or eliminating discomfort. To find a successful HT regimen, you must have confidence in your doctor and understand why you're making this decision because you may have to experiment for a while to find the right hormone regimen.

If you find yourself agreeing with some of these statements, you may want to consider HT.

✔ I have a lot of osteoporosis in my family.

✔ My mother or grandmother broke her hip.

✔ I'm miserable with these hot flashes and mood swings, and my coworkers and family members are about to put me on a rocket bound for the moon.

✔ I've been taking HT for a year now and haven't had any trouble.

✔ I'm a junk-food junkie and could never survive on rabbit food like vegetables and fruit to stay fit.

✔ My sex life is a huge problem because I'm not in the mood for it and intercourse is painful.

✔ I don't have a huge number of risk factors for osteoporosis, but I've read the statistics, and I think that I'm at greater risk for that than breast cancer.

Finding a healthy weight

A *healthy weight* is one that is associated with people who have few health problems. You can find your recommended weight by referring to weight tables published by insurance companies. Insurance companies try to figure out the weight ranges for women who live the longest. This is one of the simplest ways to determine a healthy weight.

But your very own, personal healthy weight can be fine tuned by evaluating your body fat. Body fat is the real villain in this story, not weight. To measure body fat, visit your physician or health club. Your doc (or a helpful individual at your local club) will use calipers to measure the amount of fat in several places on your body, or if she wants to be really accurate, she'll immerse you in a tub of water to see how much water you displace. A good, general rule of thumb is that healthy women have between 18 and 27 percent body fat.

Another measurement, your *body mass index* (BMI), is based on height and weight, provides a good estimation of body fat, and is easier to calculate. To determine your BMI:

1. **Multiply your height (in inches) by itself.**

2. **Divide your weight (in pounds) by the number you got in Step 1.**

3. **Multiply your answer in Step 2 by 705.**

This is your BMI. If your score is between 18.5 and 25, you're in the healthy range. If your score is between 25 and 29.9, you're in the overweight range. And if you have a BMI of 30 or higher, you're considered obese.

✔ It seems like a lot of HT options exist, so I shouldn't have a problem sticking to a schedule.

✔ I'm not big on herbal remedies to prevent or treat serious diseases.

✔ I have a good rapport with my doctor, and I'd like to give HT a try to help prevent disease.

If you still have concerns or questions, talk to your physician. Don't simply stop a therapy you're presently taking. Your medical advisor may be able to help you interpret the information you read about a study. Don't base your decision about HT — or any medication, for that matter — on TV commercials or newspaper articles.

Quitting HT

If you're taking HT when you hit menopause, it may be a good time to reevaluate your situation and consider the benefits you want to gain from hormone therapy. As you reconsider your decision, talk to your doctor. *Do not* simply stop taking HT. If you elect to quit taking HT, your doctor is the person in the best position to guide you.

Differences exist between the benefits and risks of long-term HT use and short-term HT use (refer to Tables 4-1 and 4-2 for a summary). The risks you're most worried about may not be a problem (or as big a problem) if you're taking HT for the short term — just long enough to get through the perimenopausal symptoms. With the recent study results from the Women's Health Initiative, preventing cardiovascular disease no longer seems like a good reason to begin HT. To reduce heart disease and cardiovascular risks, start by improving your diet, getting more exercise, and quitting smoking. These methods are absolutely safe and proven to reduce your risk of cardiovascular problems (including heart attack and stroke).

After you make it through the hot flashes (with or without the use of HT) and you stop having periods, it's time to consider what you want to do about preventing health problems associated with sustained, low levels of estrogen. This is a good time to reevaluate your regimen and consult with your healthcare advisor.

Chapter 5

Taking an Alternate Route: Non-Hormone Therapies

* *

In This Chapter

▶ Seasoning your therapy with herbs

▶ Healing yourself with acupuncture

▶ Subduing your symptoms with biofeedback

▶ Practicing yoga

▶ Soothing your privates with lubricants

* *

*A*t least one-third of perimenopausal and
menopausal women in the United States
use some form of *nonconventional therapy* (medical
therapies not commonly used or previously accepted
in conventional Western medicine) to treat their
symptoms.

If you're using (or considering using) nonconventional therapy, let your physician know
about the products involved because natural
supplements are still medicines — they can
alter your physiology as much as medications
from a pharmacy. (For example, some herbs

used to treat menopausal symptoms interfere with anesthesia during a surgical procedure.) Treat these nonconventional approaches as seriously as you treat other medications.

The best way to approach nontraditional therapy is to use it in conjunction with traditional medicine — each approach has benefits and problems. We devote a number of chapters in this book to hormone therapy (HT) and traditional approaches to dealing with the symptoms of perimenopause and menopause, but in this chapter, we fill in the rest of the equation. We use this chapter to introduce you to nontraditional approaches — herbs, other plant-based therapies, mind-body therapies, biofeedback, and acupuncture. But first, we review the general opinions of medical professionals and groups concerning alternative treatments that focus on herbs and other plants.

If eliminating the annoying symptoms of perimenopause were all that it took to keep women healthy (and if the alternative therapies worked reliably and effectively on all women), alternative therapies would be the best bet because they generally have fewer complications and risks when compared to hormone therapies. But staying healthy during perimenopause and menopause requires the prevention of more-serious health issues that begin when your body starts producing lower levels of estrogen.

Plowing through the Pros and Cons of Herbs

Interest in nonconventional therapy is growing. Some women enjoy taking a more holistic approach to their lives, menopause included, and others have made the choice to avoid at least some forms of conventional medicine and hormone therapy for various reasons. In this section, we detail why medical types are concerned about herbal therapies and how herbal therapies are becoming safer.

Complementary and *alternative medicines* are the names we use to refer to nonconventional therapies in this chapter. These names are just fancy ways to refer to a variety of practices and products that haven't always been considered part of conventional medicine.

 These nonconventional therapies are called *complementary* if you use them in addition to conventional medicine and *alternative* if you use them in place of conventional medicine. For example, many women who take HT also use biofeedback to further reduce stress and anxiety. In this case, biofeedback is considered complementary treatment. (For more on biofeedback, see the "Tuning in to biofeedback" section later in this chapter.) An example of an alternative therapy is using black cohosh (an herb you can read about later in this chapter) to relieve perimenopausal symptoms instead of using hormones.

Although we still use these terms, some therapies that were once considered nonconventional are sometimes incorporated into conventional medicine after years of research and success in treatment. Nonconventional courses of treatment have become so popular that the U.S. government (in the form of the National Institutes of Health; www.nih.gov) is now spending money on researching herbal and mind-body therapies like the ones we discuss in this chapter. Today, safely exploring these types of treatment is becoming easier and easier.

Taking conventional medicine's concerns into account

The biggest complaints voiced by conventional medicine concerning herb-based alternative treatments deal with the lack of scientific studies surrounding the plants. Some herbs have been studied in controlled experiments, but many have not, so researchers aren't sure whether they work any better than a sugar pill. Some therapies have been scrutinized more carefully than others, and if they work for you, that's great.

Any herb or plant therapy marketed and sold as a *medicine* in the United States must go through a U.S. Food and Drug Administration (FDA) approval process just like all other medicines (from antacids to cancer drugs). This approval process requires rigorous testing and trials. But few manufacturers of herbal therapies want to go through that process for an herb because plants can't be patented. If they spend the money to test the product and the product passes FDA muster, without a patent, competitors can copy their formula (harvest the herb and put it in a bottle). So, most manufacturers sell their products as *supplements.* Because supplements don't go through the FDA process, little proof or certification verifies that these therapies actually improve conditions as advertised and *cause no harm.*

The "cause no harm" part of the previous statement is very important. Herbs can be just as dangerous and toxic as drugs. They can interact with other medications you're currently taking. And they can produce toxic effects if taken in large quantities. Because most herbs aren't tested in recognized studies, warnings about side effects from taking an herb or too much of an herb are often sketchy, anecdotal, and not based on clinical trials. Chemicals that may be toxic are sometimes included within an herbal supplement (see the "Avoiding Problems with Plants" section later in this chapter for more info). When people ingest the herbs, they may also ingest toxic additives. The Web site of the National Center for Complementary and Alternative Medicine (www.nccam.nih.gov) has a special alert and advisory section to let you know the latest news concerning toxic effects of herbal treatments.

Conventional medicine's other complaint concerns testing for proper doses of the herbs. Many herbs are delivered to market without thorough tests of the effects of taking too large of a dose or taking the recommended dose for a long time.

When labels mention *recommended doses,* the definition of that term is often unclear. Who exactly is that dose recommended for — a person who weighs 150 pounds or a person who weighs 300 pounds? Should you take more of the supplement if your symptoms are more severe and less if they're less severe? Is there an upper threshold at which the herb becomes toxic or a lower threshold at which the herb is ineffective? Do they interfere with drugs you're currently taking?

Also, consumers often have no means of measuring the exact quantity provided in a dose. Because the FDA doesn't have to approve supplements in the United States, manufacturers are under no requirement to label the amount of drug contained in the herbal supplement.

Growing safety into herbal therapy

Before picking up a bottle of herbs off the shelf in a health-food store or incorporating herbal therapies into your life, get assistance from a qualified herbalist. Qualified herbalists are likely to have experience in predicting herbal therapies that will work for you — a great alternative to playing the eeny-meeny-miney-mo game at the health-food store. An herbalist can help you find herbs that work well together and avoid combinations that have counterproductive or toxic effects.

To find an herbalist, consult one of the many herbalist organizations. Most of these professional organizations have codes of ethics to which members must adhere and certification programs for their members. When looking for an herbalist, take all the investigative steps you would take if you were looking for a new doctor — talk to friends and interview the herbalist to find out about his or her training, practices, philosophy, and experience. An herbalist can help you put your shopping list together to make sure your therapy is as safe and effective as possible.

 Research into the safety and effectiveness of herbs is much more advanced in Germany than it is in North America, and Germany has relatively strict guidelines for regulating herbal supplements. If possible, buy herbs that have been certified in Germany because herbal therapies that meet German standards are more reliable in terms of labeling the contents and the amount of active ingredients contained in each dose.

German health authorities use the guideline of *reasonable certainty,* which means that they consider the experiences of general practitioners — not just clinical trials — in evaluating a plant drug. *The Complete German Commission E Monographs: Therapeutic Guide to Herbal Medicines* by Mark Blumenthal (Integrative Medicine Communications) is an English translation of the German "safe herb" list (the Commission E report). For more information on herbs, you can also check out *Herbal Remedies For Dummies* by Christopher Hobbs (Wiley).

Relieving Your Symptoms with Plants

Herbal treatments for the mental, emotional, and physical symptoms associated with perimenopause and menopause abound. (A lot of these herbal treatments also relieve similar premenstrual-syndrome symptoms as well.) Herbalists use a number of botanical therapies that are mild, effective, and reliable. Some therapies have been tested in clinical trials; others have proven helpful through years of use.

If you're wondering what herbal therapy can do for you, here are some of the symptoms that perimenopausal and menopausal women look to herbs to relieve and the herbs that may be effective:

- ✔ **Depression and anxiety:** *Angelica sinensis, Eleutherococcus senticosus, Ginkgo biloba, Glycyrrhiza glabra, Hypericum perforatum, Leonorus cardiaca, Panax ginseng, Verbena hastate, Withania somnifera*

- ✔ **Heart palpitations:** *Cimicifuga racemosa, Crataegus oxyacanth, Leonorus cardiaca*

- ✔ **Heavy bleeding:** *Achillea millefolium, Alchemilla vulgaris, Capsella bursa-pastoris, Myrica cerifera*

- ✔ **Hot flashes and night sweats:** *Actea racemosa, Leonorus cardiaca, Panax ginseng, Salvia officinalis*

- ✔ **Insomnia:** *Eleutherococcus senticosus, Glycyrrhiza glabra, Lavendula officinalis, Leonorus cardiac, Passiflora incarnata, Piper methysticum, Scutellaria lateriflora, Valeriana officinalis, Withania somnifera*

✔ **Memory problems:** *Bacopa moniera, Paeonia lactiflora, Panax ginseng, Gingko biloba, Rosmarinus officinalis*

✔ **Vaginal dryness:** *Actaea racemosa, Calendula officinalis, Glycyrrhiza glabra, Panax quinquefolium, Trifolium pratense*

We don't claim to be herbalists, but we do know that women in Europe and Asia have used some herbs for years to treat the symptoms of perimenopause and menopause. However, we give no advice as to dosage for a couple of reasons:

✔ **The quantity of active ingredients varies from brand to brand.**

✔ **You should always seek help from a qualified herbalist before taking herbs.**

Herbs are natural, but natural doesn't mean that they're without side effects.

Getting the Scoop on Individual Herbs

Many of the herbs used to treat perimenopausal and menopausal symptoms are phytoestrogens (*phyto* means plant, and you know what estrogen is). *Phytoestrogens* are plant estrogens — natural sources of estrogen that act as weak estrogens and seem to produce estrogen effects in menopausal women. In other words, they reduce perimenopausal and menopausal symptoms.

If you take phytoestrogens without a progestin, you're at a higher risk for endometrial cancer. Phytoestrogens are natural, but they still are mild forms of estrogen and cause your uterine lining to continue to thicken. If you use these herbs, simply mention it to your doctor. He or she can monitor your bleeding and perform tests or recommend therapy as needed. (For more information on unopposed estrogen therapy, see Chapter 3.)

Tell your doctor if you're taking any of these herbs. Some of them interfere with the effectiveness of other medicines. They're considered medicines when your doctor asks you, "What medicines are you taking?"

Ashwagandha (Withania somnifera)

Much like ginseng, eleuthero, and licorice, ashwagandha is said to reduce stress and depression and aid sleep with long-term use.

Black cohosh (Actaea racemosa syn, Cimicifuga racemosa)

Women have used black cohosh for hundreds, maybe thousands, of years. (Early Native Americans used black cohosh, and other folk medicines made use of it.) Today it's one of the more commonly used phytoestrogens in the battle against perimenopausal symptoms because it relieves hot flashes, vaginal atrophy, tension, elevated blood pressure, restless sleep, and stress.

Again, black cohosh is a phytoestrogen, so talk to your doctor before using it if you have breast cancer or if you plan on using it for more than three or four months.

If you're going to give black cohosh a try, you can find it sold under the brand name Remifemin. Remifemin is the extract approved in Germany to treat menopause, and it seems to have fewer side effects than other formulas. The German recommendation is to use it for six months or less (to avoid thickening of your endometrium).

Dong Quai (Angelica sinensis)

Also known as *tang gui,* this herb has been used for hundreds of years in traditional Chinese medicine to "strengthen the blood." Dong quai is the natural form of Coumadin (generic name: warfarin), a "blood-thinner" drug doctors often prescribe for women who have *arrhythmia* (irregular heart beat) because it dilates the blood vessels and decreases clotting to improve blood flow to your heart. It also seems to eliminate hot flashes.

Possible drawbacks? Dong quai reduces blood clotting, so if you're having surgery be sure to let your doctor know beforehand that you've been using this herb. You should stop using it two weeks before surgery. Also, don't use dong quai if you've had unexplained vaginal bleeding. Try to avoid aspirin and other drugs that serve to thin your blood while using this herb.

Ginkgo (Gingko biloba)

Here's one that's been in the news quite a bit. This herb is said to improve your memory and feeling of well-being, and one study of 200 women showed that it increased sexual desire.

But don't use it with abandon. Ginkgo reduces blood clotting (it thins your blood), so be sure to let your doctor know that you're using this herb. If you're scheduled to undergo an operation, quit taking ginko at least two weeks before surgery. And don't take it if you're taking other blood thinners such as the drug Coumadin (or the herb dong quai).

Ginseng (Panax ginseng,
Panax quinqafolium)

People all over the world consume ginseng to increase vitality, improve memory, relieve anxiety, and kick-start low libido. Historically, menopausal women have used ginseng to relieve depression, fatigue, memory lapses, and low libido. It doesn't seem to raise your estrogen levels or cause your endometrium to thicken as some of the phytoestrogens tend to do.

You have to be careful about using ginseng if you're taking other types of medication for depression or anxiety. It's been known to cause mania when combined with certain antidepressant medications.

Kava (Piper methysticum)

Herbalists use kava to reduce anxiety and chronic pain and to promote sleep and relaxation. However, even herbalists recognize a need for further tests to determine if this herb is potentially toxic to the liver.

This herb may be harmful to your liver. Talk to your doctor if you choose to take it.

Motherwort (Leonorus cardiaca)

The Chinese have used motherwort for a long time. Western herbalists make use of it to treat menopausal anxiety, insomnia, heart palpitations, and vaginal atrophy.

Peony (Paeonia lactiflora)

Peony helps dilate the blood vessels so that blood flows more smoothly through your cardiovascular system. Some folks claim that it also improves your mental focus and reduces mental lapses.

Red clover (Trifolium pratense)

Menopausal women often find that this herb, historically used to treat skin and breathing problems, relieves vaginal dryness and lowers their LDL (bad cholesterol) levels while increasing their HDL (the good stuff) levels. Red clover contains *isoflavones* (the chemicals that make phytoestrogens work like estrogen), so it acts as a mild estrogen.

As with all phytoestrogens, don't use red clover if you have breast cancer.

Sage (Salvia officinalis)

Sage is said to relieve hot flashes, but the claim hasn't been widely researched.

Saint John's wort (Hypericum perforatum)

The popularity of Saint John's wort for treating depression has grown tremendously in recent years, but people have used this herb since the Middle Ages. During perimenopause and menopause, women use it to treat mild depression. Although many published reports show that Saint John's wort does work, how it works is a question that we don't have an answer for.

Saint John's wort can cause sensitivity to light. It also interferes with a variety of other medications, so as with any herb, tell your doctor that you're taking it.

Soy

Soy is a plant estrogen (phytoestrogen), so it has the same pluses and problems as other phytoestrogens. It's reported to relieve hot flashes, interrupted sleep, anxiety, and other perimenopausal symptoms. However, too much soy has the same effect as unopposed estrogen (unfettered thickening of the uterine lining).

Although many advertisements for soy products point to the health of women in Japan and China as evidence that they work, women in these cultures start eating soy early in life, and they eat mostly fermented-soy products, such as *miso* (soybean paste) and *tempeh* (a cheese-like soybean food), rather than soy-protein drinks and milk. But studies have shown that soy can clean up your blood by reducing your total cholesterol, LDL cholesterol (bad cholesterol), triglycerides, and blood pressure while raising your HDL (good cholesterol) levels.

Vitex (Vitex agnus castus)

Vitex, or *chaste tree,* acts like progesterone by helping to reduce perimenopausal stress and depression. (Some women have found that it does just the opposite, but reports of vitex causing stress and depression are rare.) Because it acts like progesterone, vitex may help stabilize the uterine lining. Herbalists say that it's safe for long-term use.

Avoiding Problems with Plants

As we state throughout this chapter, just because herbs are natural doesn't mean they're safe. People get into trouble with herbs because they don't realize that herbs are drugs that produce both positive and negative effects. Some people with certain medical conditions are more susceptible to side effects associated with some herbs. For example, women with cardiovascular disease should be careful with herbs because the containers don't necessarily carry any warning. Here are some other things to look out for when using herbs:

- ✔ **Some herbs can damage your liver causing chronic hepatitis or acute liver injury.** These herbs include chaparral, coltsfoot, comfrey, germander, Gordolobo yerba tea, mate tea, pennyroyal oil (also known as squaw mint), and many others.

- ✔ **Therapies that contain the active ingredient** *mefanamic acid* **can cause liver and kidney damage (and sometimes your kidneys quit functioning altogether, which spells trouble).**

- ✔ **Any herb or supplement that includes** *ephedra* **or caffeine is dangerous for women with high blood pressure or cardiovascular disease.** (The Chinese herb *mahuang* is the same thing as ephedra.) Unfortunately, caffeine is often added to tonics and supplements without being listed on the label.

If you feel heart palpitations or anxiety with any herbal therapy, stop using it immediately.

Getting Touchy about Acupuncture

Acupuncture is a form of Chinese medicine in which an acupuncturist inserts needles into specific points along critical energy paths in your body. For the doubters out there, acupuncture isn't all that far out. Asian doctors have successfully performed surgeries using acupuncture as the anesthesia.

Acupuncture stimulates your body's ability to resist or overcome menopausal symptoms by correcting energy imbalances. Acupuncture also prompts your body to produce chemicals that decrease or eliminate pain and discomfort.

Acupuncturists place fine needles into your body, which affect your *chi* — your life-force energy that travels through pathways in your body that are called *meridians*. Acupuncturists have mapped out the meridians and specific points along the meridians in the human body, so they know where to place the needle given your specific symptoms. You tell the acupuncturist your symptoms — heavy bleeding, headaches, and hot flashes, for example — and he or she knows exactly how to place the needles to relieve your discomfort.

Acupuncture is recognized as a legitimate form of complementary or alternative medicine, and many insurance plans cover this type of therapy. If you're interested in trying this therapy, find a qualified specialist. Many states regulate and license acupuncturists, so you can probably get names of licensed acupuncturists from your state department of health.

Soothing Symptoms with Relaxation Therapies

Stress can be great if it motivates you to do your best — like in a race. But, if you're continually stressed out, stress can actually do physical damage to your mind and body. It can lead to excessive eating, sleeplessness, anxiety, depression, and irritability. (Do any of these symptoms sound familiar — as in perimenopausal and menopausal symptoms?) Continued stress can also affect your immune system, making you more susceptible to cancer, hypertension, heart problems, and headaches — the medical concerns women worry about after menopause.

Take a look at some of these nonmedical therapies that can help you relax and reduce the stress in your life. With stress, like Brylcreem, "A little dab will do you."

Tuning in to biofeedback

Biofeedback relies on the interconnectedness of the mind and body. Back in the 1600s, to appease the Christian church, medical pioneers drew an artificial line between the body and the spirit and told religious leaders that medicine would concern itself only with the physical body. Centuries later, Western medicine is trying to reunite the mind and body in their proper interconnected context in order to make our approaches to healing more comprehensive.

Biofeedback has been around since the 1960s, but it uses some of the mind-body lessons taught by ancient martial arts. The biggest difference between biofeedback and the martial arts is technology. Biofeedback uses monitoring instruments to provide you with physiological information (feedback) — information you otherwise wouldn't be aware of. By watching the monitoring device, and through trial and error, you learn to adjust your thinking and mental attitudes to control bodily processes that folks used to think were involuntary. Using biofeedback, some people learn to control their blood pressure, temperature, gastrointestinal functioning, and brainwave activity.

Some of the menopause-related conditions you can treat with biofeedback are

- ✔ Hypertension
- ✔ Migraine headaches
- ✔ Sleep difficulties
- ✔ Stress
- ✔ Urinary incontinence

Getting your yoga groove on

Now here's a great way to kill two birds with one stone. Yoga can help you improve your flexibility (something that starts decreasing after you've been on this planet for about 35 years) and relieve stress. Staying flexible is an important part of balance; so being flexible reduces your chance of falling and breaking a bone. Reducing stress improves your immunity by helping you avoid disease and also improve your mental outlook.

Yoga is also a great way to keep your bones strong and improve your muscle tone. Yoga combines breathing, meditation, and stretching techniques to help strengthen bones and muscles and improve posture, breathing, oxygen flow, relaxation, and overall health and vitality. Take a class or grab a book — many different forms of yoga are out there, and it's great for women of all ages.

Slip Sliding Away with Topical Treatments

Many perimenopausal and menopausal women experience *vaginal atrophy* (drying and thinning of the vagina). You can treat this condition in several ways without using hormone therapy.

You can buy lubricants without a prescription in the grocery store that will help relieve the day-to-day discomfort of vaginal dryness. Replens is one of the more popular brands of lubricants and has shown to be as effective as vaginal estrogen cream in relieving vaginal dryness in tests. Replens comes in a tube with an applicator. You simply fill the applicator, insert the tube into your vagina, and press the applicator. You do this once a week.

In addition to over-the-counter lubricants, some of the herbs we discuss in this chapter also relieve vaginal dryness.

If vaginal atrophy is causing painful intercourse, we have a prescription-free solution for you. A number of lubricants are designed to help you get slippery. In fact, you may find that sex is more fun when you "butter up" than it was before. K-Y Jelly has been around for years. Hospitals and doctors' offices use it for lubricating thermometers when taking temperatures rectally and for many other purposes. It also works well as a lubricant before intercourse. Astroglide is another terrific product that can make you more slippery. You can rub all of these products on your vagina prior to intercourse.

Chapter 6

Treating Conditions without Hormone Therapy

* *

In This Chapter

▶ Beefing up your bones without estrogen

▶ Heading toward a healthy heart without hormones

* *

*P*rolonged periods of low estrogen levels can promote bone deterioration and cardiovascular conditions. Although many women choose to use hormone therapy (HT) to prevent these issues, other medications and therapies that directly treat these issues are available. The treatments we discuss in this chapter are targeted to specific conditions or diseases. Hormone therapy tries to treat these conditions indirectly by adjusting hormone levels. Whether or not you use hormones, you can use the treatments we cover in this chapter. Some of the treatments are medications; others are lifestyle choices.

Battling Bone Loss and Osteoporosis with Medication

One of the best ways to avoid *osteoporosis* (brittle bone disease) is to start out with strong, healthy bones. You can accomplish this feat by getting plenty of calcium and vitamins D and K in your diet during childhood, adolescence, and early adulthood. Of course, hindsight is 20/20, and it may be too late at this point in your life to start developing healthy bone mass. (But it may not be too late for the young women in your life, so spread the word.) Fear not: In the following sections, we outline some other ways to improve the health of your bones during menopause without using HT.

A number of drugs can help preserve bone density. The drugs we mention in this chapter, taken in combination with a healthy diet and an exercise program, can slow the rate of bone loss and, in many cases, actually increase bone density over time.

Talking bisphosphonates

A group of drugs called *bisphosphonates* are the most effective medications for halting and reversing bone loss in menopausal women. These drugs work by slowing the destruction part *(resorption)* of the bone-maintenance process. The following list contains some examples of bisphosphonates. Unless otherwise noted, we list the drugs by their brand names followed by the generic names in parentheses.

Fosamax (alendronate): This medication is one of the most commonly used bisphosphonates. Approved by the Food and Drug Administration for use in the United States in 1995, Fosamax prevents bone material from breaking down, and it actually builds stronger bones. When you include this medication as part of a healthy lifestyle (including enough calcium and regular exercise), you can cut your risk of fracture in half.

Like all medications, Fosamax comes with some rules. You have to

- ✔ **Take it first thing in the morning on a completely empty stomach.** You may have to adjust your morning schedule if you like to hop out of bed and into the coffee pot.

- ✔ **Take it with a full glass of water.** Don't substitute coffee, juice, cola, or anything else. Use plain water.

- ✔ **Remain upright after taking it.** Sorry, but you can't go back to bed. If you don't remain upright after you take it, Fosamax can cause a reflux type of reaction in which you have a burning sensation in your esophagus.

- ✔ **Wait for an hour after taking it before you eat breakfast.** Actually the longer you wait to eat or drink anything, the better your body absorbs the medication. Waiting two hours before eating is even better than waiting just one. If you wait two hours, your body absorbs nearly 70 percent of the drug, but if you only wait 30 minutes, the number drops to about 46 percent. If you eat when you take Fosamax, you won't absorb enough of the medication to help your bones.

Fosamax comes in once-a-day and once-a-week pill form. It presents very few side effects when you take it correctly. Women who are taking hormone therapy can use this drug to get even more protection from fracture.

Actonel (risedronate): This bisphosphonate received approval for use in the United States for preventing and treating osteoporosis in early 2000. Actonel is supposed to have fewer gastrointestinal side effects than Fosamax presents, and it has a slightly better track record in reducing the risk of fracture (65 percent reduction in the risk of fracture for Actonel versus 47 percent for Fosamax). Actonel comes in once-a-day or once-a-week pill form. You can take this medication even if you take hormone therapy.

Introducing calcitonin

Miacalcin (calcitonin) is a nasal spray that uses a different technique to slow down bone loss than the bisphosphonates use. Calcitonin is actually a hormone that occurs naturally in your body. It helps regulate your calcium levels by slowing the rate of bone deterioration. It also relieves bone pain caused by osteoporosis.

The rules with this stuff are a bit simpler but still pretty specific. You use one squirt in one nostril per day, alternating nostrils on a daily basis. (Is this a cruel joke or what? Don't the Miacalcin bigwigs know that menopausal women often experience memory lapses?) Calcitonin isn't quite as effective at preventing bone loss as the bisphosphonates, but it may reduce the pain of existing spinal fractures.

Considering fluoride

Fluoride stimulates bone building, but the bone it builds seems to be brittle. All the bisphosphonates treat osteoporosis by slowing the natural bone destruction process, but fluoride works on the other side of the bone-maintenance equation by aiding the formation of new bone.

Although fluoride increases bone density, it doesn't reduce fractures. After reading that statement, you may be thinking, "What good is thick bone if it's not

strong?" Good question. That's why fluoride isn't nor-
mally used to treat osteoporosis. Some new research
is being conducted using slow-release fluoride along
with calcium supplements to see if stronger bones
can be built. Stay tuned for more.

Controlling Cardiovascular Disease

Cardiovascular disease includes conditions that affect
the blood, blood vessels, or heart (otherwise known as
the cardiovascular system). Controlling cardiovascular
disease is the big one. Reducing the risks of cardiovascular disease was thought to be one of the biggest
benefits of HT, but the results of the Women's Health
Initiative study have called all that into question.

The risks of cardiovascular disease are high for
women after menopause — nearly one out of every
two women in the United States will die of some type
of cardiovascular disease. Given the high incidence
of cardiovascular disease in women over 50 and the
controversy over whether hormone therapy increases
or decreases your risk, you *really* need to put some
thought into how to keep your blood, blood vessels,
and heart healthy for the next 40 or 50 years. In the following sections, we provide you with some strategies.

Reducing your risk of heart attack with drugs

Half of all heart attacks occur in people with normal
cholesterol levels, so a healthy cholesterol profile
doesn't mean you're out of the woods. Of course, the
other side of that story is that half of all heart attacks
occur in people with lousy cholesterol profiles. So try

to maintain a healthy diet and exercise program and take your cholesterol medication if your doctor recommends it.

Arteriosclerosis (clogged arteries) isn't the only problem that triggers a heart attack. Many other conditions can lead to a heart attack as well:

- ✔ Angina (blood vessel spasms)
- ✔ Arrhythmia (irregular heart beat)
- ✔ Blood clots
- ✔ High blood pressure

To reduce your risk of heart attack, be sure to maintain a healthy diet, exercise regularly, and take the medication your doctor prescribes to treat high cholesterol and any of these cardiovascular conditions. The following are other medications used to control or prevent heart attack:

- ✔ **ACE inhibitors:** Docs often use ACE inhibitors on people who have recently had a heart attack and who have heart failure or decreased function of the left ventricle. If used within 24 hours of the start of heart-attack symptoms, ACE inhibitors can keep you from dying of the heart attack and prevent heart failure stemming from the heart attack. The "ACE" part stands for *angiotensin-converting enzyme* — we threw that in here just in case you're a big fan of medical terms.

- ✔ **Aspirin:** Recently, people have started paying a whole lot of renewed attention to this trusted pain reliever. The buzz surrounds aspirin's ability to lower the risk of heart attack when taken every day. Aspirin performs this function by keeping your *platelets* (special blood cells responsible for clotting) from sticking together too much and forming blood clots unnecessarily. Aspirin is what's known as an *anticoagulant* (it keeps your blood from coagulating, or clotting). If your body starts forming clots too readily, the clots can clog your blood vessels and lead to heart attack or stroke. If you have angina, your doctor may recommend aspirin to avoid a heart attack. Or if you've already had a heart attack, your doctor may recommend that you take aspirin daily to avoid another attack.

Warning: Even though aspirin is an over-the-counter medication, it can have dangerous side effects. Read the warning label on the bottle and discuss possible side effects with your doctor. And even though preventing blood clots with aspirin can help you avoid a heart attack, blood clotting is an important bodily function that stops you from bleeding if you cut yourself or have surgery. Be sure to tell your doctor that you're taking aspirin regularly if you're facing surgery.

✔ **Coumadin:** You may see this drug referred to by its generic name, warfarin. Coumadin is another drug doctors use to prevent blood from clotting. But unlike aspirin, it's a prescription drug. Coumadin is more effective than aspirin in preventing blood clots, so you must use caution and have your blood monitored regularly when taking it. Women who have angina or who have irregular heartbeats often take this medication to help move blood more fluidly through the vessels.

✔ **Thrombolytics:** Doctors give a member of this class of drugs to patients having a heart attack because of a blood clot. Thrombolytics can dissolve a clot and restore blood flow to the heart. These drugs must be administered within six hours of the heart attack (before heart tissue begins to die from lack of oxygen) to be effective.

✔ **Vasodilators:** These drugs help blood vessels relax and *dilate* (widen) so that your heart doesn't have to work as hard to get oxygen-rich blood into the heart muscle. *Nitroglycerin* is a common vasodilator given to women who suffer from angina. Take these drugs as directed by your doctor.

Treating high blood pressure with drugs

A variety of drugs are available today that treat *hypertension* (high blood pressure). They fall into two main categories:

✔ **Beta-blockers:** A number of different types of beta-blockers are sold under a variety of brand names. These drugs reduce your heart rate and blood pressure. Sometimes doctors also prescribe them to treat angina.

✔ **Calcium channel blockers:** These drugs reduce your heart's oxygen requirements, increase the blood supply to your heart, and lower blood pressure. They can prevent coronary artery spasms if you have angina.

Keeping your blood lean and mean with drugs

Blood that's high in LDL cholesterol (the bad stuff) and triglycerides encourages the fat and cholesterol to build up in the lining of your blood vessels, which leads to *arteriosclerosis* (hardening of the arteries) and can eventually cause a heart attack.

But some medications can lower bad cholesterol (LDL)
and triglyceride levels and raise good cholesterol
(HDL) levels. These medications are called *antilipemic
drugs* because they help moderate your lipid levels
(cholesterol and triglycerides). Here's what the
National Cholesterol Education Program recommends
to keep your cholesterol levels in check and to keep
your cardiovascular system healthy:

- ✔ Get your blood cholesterol levels checked
  every year (total cholesterol, LDL, HDL, and
  triglycerides).

- ✔ Visit your doctor regularly to assess your risk of
  cardiovascular problems.

- ✔ Read the labels on your foods and choose foods
  that are low in saturated fat and cholesterol.

- ✔ Keep your weight in check.

- ✔ Exercise regularly.

- ✔ Don't smoke, and avoid second-hand smoke.

If changes in your diet, activity level, and lifestyle
don't improve your cholesterol levels, your doctor
may recommend medication to improve your cholesterol profile. Several types of drugs are available to
lower cholesterol:

- ✔ **Bile acid sequestrants:** These drugs lower LDL
  levels and can be used alone or in combination
  with statin drugs.

- ✔ **Fibric acids:** Fibric acids lower LDL levels a bit
  but usually are used to treat high-triglyceride
  and low-HDL levels.

- ✔ **Nicotinic acids:** These babies lower LDL and
  triglyceride levels and raise HDL levels.

- ✔ **Statins:** These drugs are very effective in lowering LDL levels.

Your doctor is the only person who can determine whether cholesterol-lowering drugs are
right for you and which type of drugs can meet
your needs.

Living a hearty lifestyle

Here's a simple fact: Study after study has shown that
smoking absolutely increases your risk of cardiovascular problems because it promotes the buildup of
fat and cholesterol in your arteries and increases the
formation of blood clots that can cause heart attacks.
Eliminating smoking is a good way to lower your risk
of cardiovascular disease. Your risk begins to drop
immediately after you quit. By your tenth anniversary
of beginning a smoke-free life, your risk of cardiovascular disease is similar to that of a woman who never
smoked.

Smoking isn't the only enemy of cardiovascular
health. Weight matters. Gaining more than 12 to
18 pounds after age 18 increases your risk of
coronary heart disease, and your risk becomes
greater as you gain more weight. If you've gained
40 or more pounds since your 18th birthday,
you've doubled your risk of heart disease. If you
want to look at the connection in a more positive
light, you'll be glad to know that your cholesterol
drops 25 points with every 10 pounds you lose.

A life full of anger, anxiety, depression, and isola-
tion also increases your risk of cardiovascular
disease. If one or more of these emotional conditions rule your life, it's not healthy, especially for
your cardiovascular system. Having a network of
friends or relatives who can offer you emotional
support can lower your risk of cardiovascular
disease. Try meditation or physical activity to

reduce anger, depression, and anxiety. You may want to share your symptoms with a healthcare provider in order to begin treating them.

Picking a heart-healthy diet

The National Cancer Institute recommends eating at least five fruits and vegetables each day to reduce your risk of heart disease (and cancer). "Get five to survive, but nine is divine" is a slogan used by the Cooper Institute, one of the most prestigious preventative-health institutions in the world. The institute is talking about the number of servings of fruits and vegetables you should consume *each day.* That means you need to spend less time in front of the dairy case and more time in the produce section at the grocery store. Five to nine servings of fruits and vegetables sounds like a lot, but meeting this goal is actually pretty easy.

Chapter 7

Ten (or So) Medical Tests for Menopausal Women

*T*his chapter lists some basic health tests that help doctors identify diseases and other problems in their early stages — when they're more treatable. *Early detection* is the key to successful treatment of nearly every disease that affects menopausal women.

Avoiding the tests doesn't mean that you can avoid the related diseases, so visit your doctors regularly and follow through with their recommendations.

Pelvic Exam and Pap Smear

No one likes to put her feet in the stirrups and her privates in the saddle every year, but doing so surely helps you avoid some nasty problems down the line. You should have an annual gynecological exam. The gynecologist will check your female organs including your breasts, your vaginal tissue, your cervix, and your uterus. Your gynecologist will also perform a *Pap smear* to test for cervical cancer every year.

If you've had a complete hysterectomy for benign reasons, you should have a pelvic exam and Pap smear (to check for noncancerous medical issues) every year for three years; after that, the Pap can be done once every three years. However, you still need a breast and pelvic exam every year.

Rectal Exam

Everyone squirms when this exam is the subject at hand. Everybody hates it, but the risks of postponing a rectal exam can be quite devastating to you and your loved ones. Regular rectal exams can help detect problems early — when they can be easily and painlessly treated.

Part of this test is a *digital exam* in which the doctor checks your organs for signs of disease. The doctor inserts a gloved finger into your rectum to evaluate the health of your tissues. Keep in mind that the long-term benefits greatly outweigh the short-term unpleasantness of the procedure. And also remember that your doctor *chose* this field of medicine.

The other part of this exam is a *fecal occult test,* which enables doctors to check whether you have blood in your stool. This part of the test is necessary because the presence of blood can be an indication of problems, such as cancer, in your colon.

You should have a rectal exam once a year during your annual gynecological physical, especially after age 50.

Colonoscopy

Colon cancer is a form of cancer that progresses very slowly and is readily treatable. But it's the third leading cause of cancer deaths among American women. No one likes the test — it's that simple. And women avoid discussing the issue until they have symptoms. The problem is that patients very often don't experience any symptoms until the disease is in an advanced stage — a point when successful treatment is much more difficult.

While performing a colonoscopy, your doctor can find and remove precancerous polyps (doctors know them as *adenomatous polyps*) before they have a chance of becoming cancerous. The night before your colonoscopy, you drink a potion that helps clean out your colon. While you're under the influence of a light sedative, the doctor inserts a flexible scope into your colon that allows her to view the colon walls in search of polyps or other unhealthy tissue. If she finds a polyp, she can remove it and send it to the lab for analysis. Lab analysis determines whether the polyp is benign or precancerous.

Want to cut your risk of colon cancer by one-third? All you have to do is regularly schedule (and go through with) a colonoscopy. If you're over 50, have a colonoscopy every five years — more often if you have polyps.

Bone-Density Screening

Your best bet is to have at least one bone-density screening before you're menopausal. When you're 40, visit your doctor and get a baseline bone-density screening. The results provide your doctors with something to compare future screenings to. If you show signs of bone loss in this or subsequent tests, you'll have bone screenings every two years.

If your family has a history of osteoporosis (your sister, mother, or grandmother have osteoporosis), get a baseline bone-density screening when you're in your late thirties.

If you've never had a bone screening and you're over 40, talk to your doctor about your options.

Mammogram

Early detection is the key to reducing your risk of breast cancer, so you should begin getting annual mammograms when you're 40 years old with a base-line taken at age 35. If your mother or sister has had breast cancer, get your first mammogram even earlier, when you're 30.

 The American Cancer Society recommends that you get a mammogram every one to two years after age 40 and every year after you turn 50. Other groups advise less frequent mammo-grams. In our opinion, annual mammograms are your best bet even if scientists are still debating the merits of a yearly regimen.

Cholesterol Screening

A cholesterol screening checks your total cholesterol, *LDL cholesterol* (bad cholesterol), *HDL cholesterol* (good cholesterol), and *triglycerides* (another form of fat found in your blood) and computes your choles-terol ratio. Take this simple blood test every five years. You should take it when you're fasting — nothing to eat or drink for 12 hours before the test. If your doctor identifies problems with your cholesterol or triglyceride levels or you have a history of high blood pressure, diabetes, thyroid problems, or obesity, your doctor may want to screen you more frequently.

Fasting Blood-Glucose Test

Adult-onset diabetes can lead to coronary heart disease, so you want to diagnose this problem early. Begin having your blood sugar *(glucose)* tested when you're 20 and repeat the test every three to five years — more frequently if you experience problems. The blood-glucose test is a simple blood test administered after you've had nothing to eat or drink for 12 hours (that's where the *fasting* part of the name comes from). You can also screen for diabetes by checking for sugar in your urine.

Thyroid Screening

The symptoms of thyroid problems and the symptoms of menopause can be quite similar. Get your first thyroid screening at age 35. The screening measures your levels of thyroid-stimulating hormone (THS) and thyroid antibodies.

CA 125 Test

Doctors don't routinely perform this blood test during your annual gynecological exam. But you may want to take it if you have a family history of ovarian cancer or if you're having abdominal bloating or pain or other symptoms that evade diagnosis or don't respond to other treatments. Levels of the CA 125 antigen often rise with the presence of ovarian cancer, endometriosis, ovarian cysts, fibroids, and even the early stages of pregnancy.

This exam isn't considered a diagnostic test for ovarian cancer because higher levels of CA 125 don't necessarily indicate ovarian cancer, and sometimes, levels don't rise if you have ovarian cancer. But high levels of CA 125 can be an early warning of ovarian cancer and cause your doctor to pursue additional tests until ovarian cancer can be ruled out.

Ovarian Hormone Screening

Out of necessity, the standard practice for prescribing hormone therapy is a method of trial and error — a "try-this-regimen-and-let-me-know-how-you-feel" kind of approach. Everybody processes hormones differently, so the amount of hormone in a medication isn't the amount that reaches your bloodstream. For example, the same form of estrogen may affect two women differently. And your body may respond better to some estrogens than to others.

The key to what "works" and what doesn't is the amount of *estradiol* (the active form of estrogen) your body produces in response to the estrogen you're taking. The only accurate way to know how much estradiol you're churning out is to draw blood and analyze it for hormone levels. (Saliva tests are available, but they're less accurate.)

That said, the majority of doctors stick with the standard dosing formulas and do the trial-and-error thing until you tell them you're feeling better. We just want you to know that an alternative (ovarian hormone screening) is available and a bit more objective.

Estradiol levels below 90 pg/ml result in the typical hot flashes, interrupted sleep, mood swings, and other annoying perimenopausal symptoms. If your levels drop below 80 or 90 pg/ml, you risk suffering from bone loss and cardiovascular issues. So the key is to get your estradiol levels up to 90 or 100 pg/ml after menopause.

 Sometime during your 20s or 30s, you should have a hormone screening to check your pre-menopausal baseline levels of estrogen, progesterone, and testosterone at two points in your menstrual cycle — Day 1 or 2 of your cycle and then again at around Day 18 (assuming a 28-day cycle). The technician draws some blood and sends it to a lab for analysis. The results give you an idea of your typical hormone levels prior to menopause.

But never having had a baseline drawn is okay — you can still benefit from ovarian hormone screening. If you've been experimenting with hormone therapy and want to get off the roller coaster, you may want to ask your doctor to check out your current hormone levels to see how effectively your therapy is working.

Stress Test

You may think that your life has been one big stress test, but actually, a stress test is a legitimate medical procedure. A stress test is basically an electrocardiogram (EKG) that a technician performs while you walk on a treadmill. You may have had an EKG in the past to qualify for life insurance or as part of an annual exam. The purpose of the test is to see how your heart responds to the stress of exercise. If you're overweight, have high blood pressure, or experience chest pain or shortness of breath with mild exertion, your doctor may suggest a stress test. Your doctor may also perform a stress test to check out your heart before you begin a new exercise program.

The procedure is simple. A technician sticks some electrical wires on your chest to record the electrical activity in your heart. This information tells the doctor if your heart is getting enough oxygen or if it's been damaged. To stress your heart, you walk on a special treadmill while you're plugged into the EKG.

You should take a stress test if your doctor suspects that you have coronary artery disease; otherwise, get a baseline reading at 40 and then take the test every three to five years.

The risk of heart attack rises after menopause, so don't overlook the importance of checking out the health of your heart.

Diet, Health & Fitness Titles from For Dummies

For Dummies books help keep you healthy and fit. Whatever
your health & fitness needs, turn to Dummies books first.

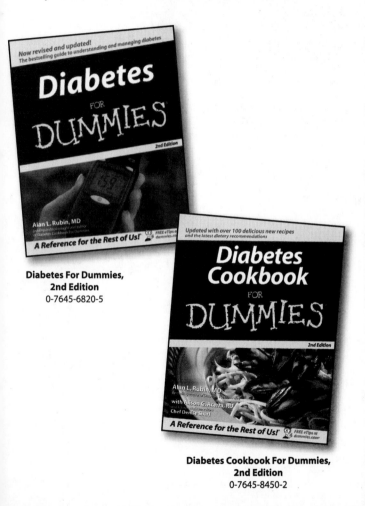

**Diabetes For Dummies,
2nd Edition**
0-7645-6820-5

**Diabetes Cookbook For Dummies,
2nd Edition**
0-7645-8450-2

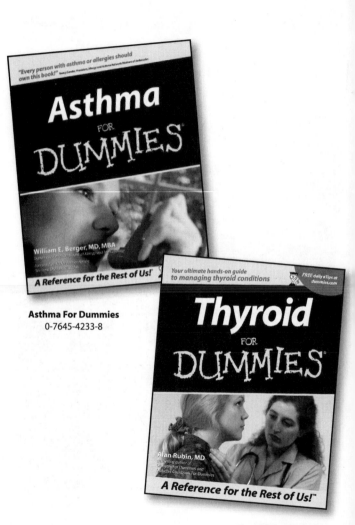

Asthma For Dummies
0-7645-4233-8

Thyroid For Dummies
0-7645-5385-2

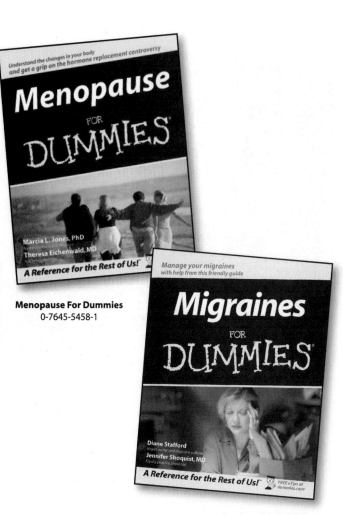

Menopause For Dummies
0-7645-5458-1

Migraines For Dummies
0-7645-5485-9

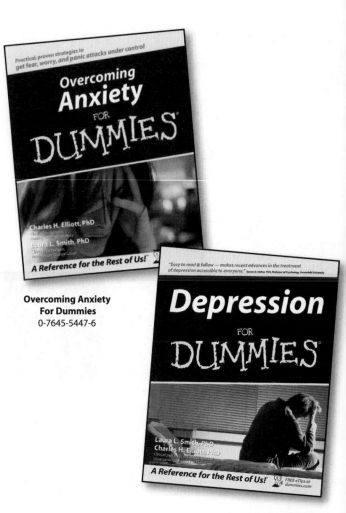

**Overcoming Anxiety
For Dummies**
0-7645-5447-6

Depression For Dummies
0-7645-3900-0